a **taste** for health

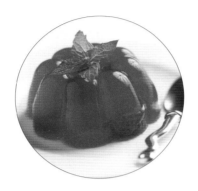

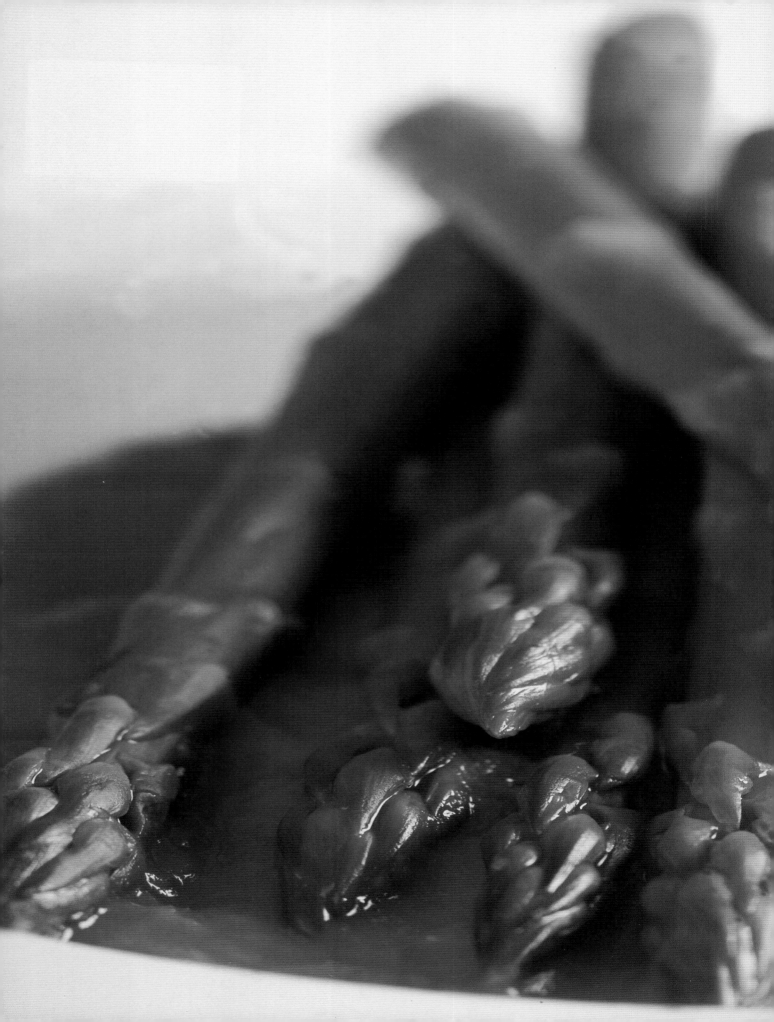

a **taste** for health

Pat Barton & Magdaleen van Wyk

HUMAN & ROUSSEAU

Cape Town   Pretoria   Johannesburg

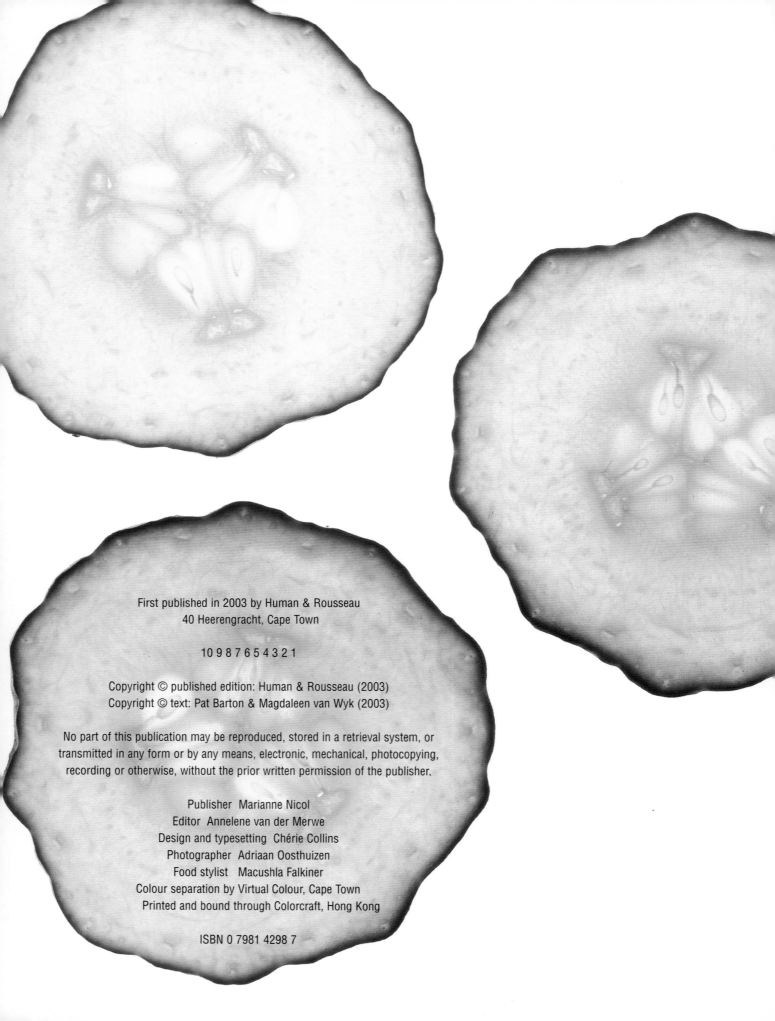

First published in 2003 by Human & Rousseau
40 Heerengracht, Cape Town

10 9 8 7 6 5 4 3 2 1

Publisher Marianne Nicol
Editor Annelene van der Merwe
Design and typesetting Chérie Collins
Photographer Adriaan Oosthuizen
Food stylist Macushla Falkiner
Colour separation by Virtual Colour, Cape Town
Printed and bound through Colorcraft, Hong Kong

ISBN 0 7981 4298 7

contents

healthy living

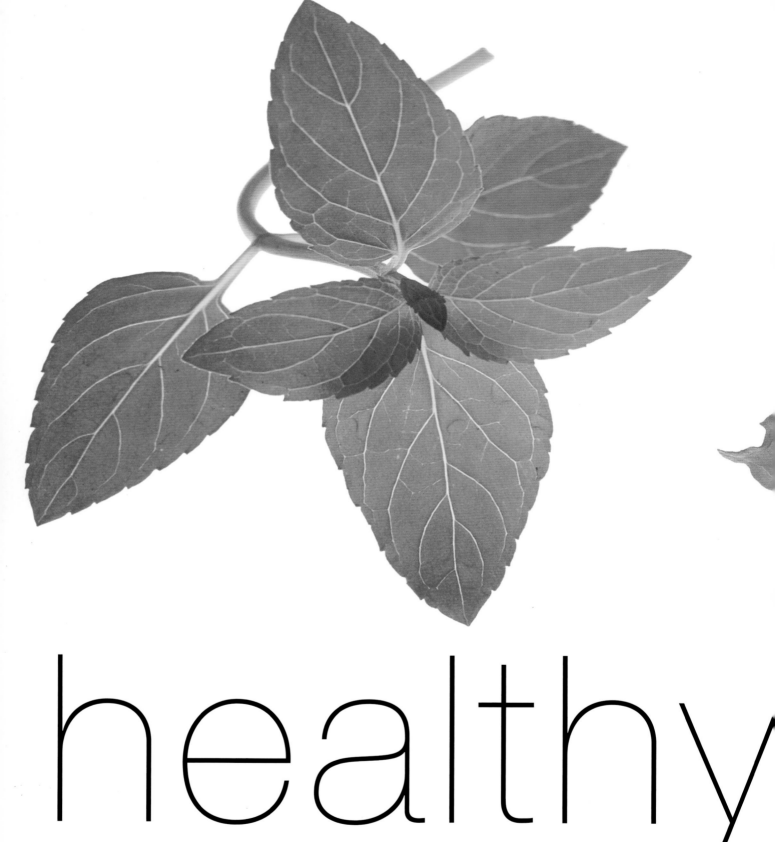

healthy

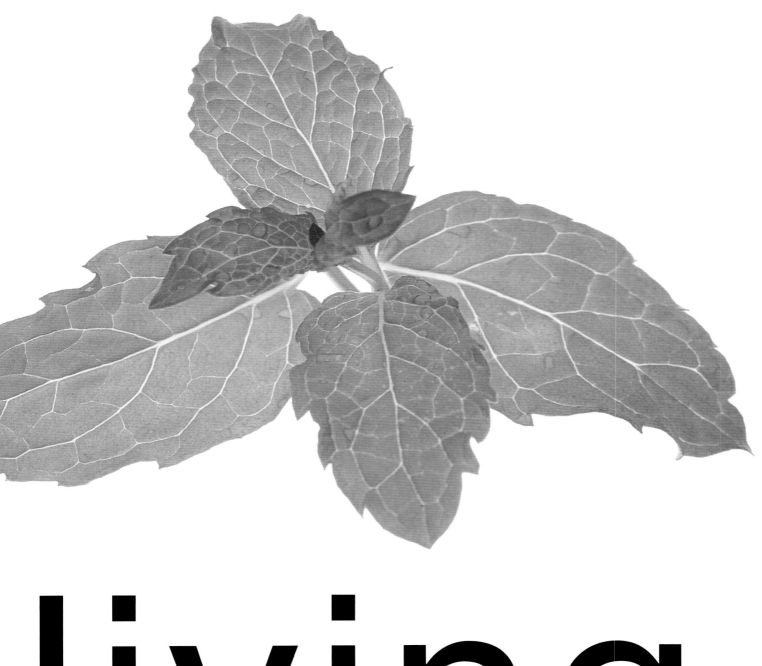

living

Nutrition and a healthy lifestyle

The old adage 'you are what you eat', is largely true – good nutrition is indeed the basis of good health. Not only does it help heal the sick, protect the aged and build up strong young bodies; it is also what we should all strive to achieve for a long and healthy life.

The effects of poor nutrition are often not seen in strong young people; it's only later, mainly from middle age onwards, that problems such as heart disease, high blood pressure and cancer take hold … all of which might have been prevented by healthy eating.

What *A taste for health* attempts to do is provide guidelines for optimal nutrition – and therefore optimal health – for all of us. This means not only information on eating healthily, but also on therapeutic nutrition. While it does not attempt to be a medical reference, it is hoped that *A taste for health* will guide you to a better understanding of some of the more common illnesses that require a special diet.

What makes *A taste for health* unique is the way it combines the science of nutrition with tasty, eye-appealing recipes, making it a joy to prepare and savour dishes that you know are good for you. Here, too, people on special diets will find tempting recipes that use ingredients they're allowed to eat. Information on how to use the recipes is given on page 62.

NUTRIENTS, METABOLISM AND ENERGY

Because our bodies have only a limited capacity for storing nutrients (except those they store as fat), we need to replenish most nutrients daily, in balanced quantities, throughout our lifetimes. Not everyone needs these nutrients in the same quantities; for example, growing children and pregnant women need more of some nutrients than the rest of us.

All the essential nutrients – proteins, carbohydrates, fats, minerals and vitamins – that our bodies need are provided by a diet composed of meat, fish, legumes, milk and dairy products, eggs, fruit, vegetables, cereals and whole-grain products.

As foods are used (burned, or metabolised) in the body, they provide energy which makes possible our daily activities, as well as vital functions such as breathing, cardiovascular activity and the maintenance of muscle tone. The energy value of foods is expressed in kilojoules (kJ).

Only three nutrients yield energy when metabolised: carbohydrates, fats and protein. Carbohydrates and proteins each yield 17 kJ per gram, while fats yield 37 kJ per gram. Foods differ in kilojoule value because the quantity of carbohydrates, protein, fats and water they contain, differs. For example, because water contains no kilojoules, foods that contain a high proportion of water, such as lettuce, spinach and tomatoes, are low in kilojoules.

We differ from one another in our energy needs, which depend on age, size, gender, and activity levels. But regardless of what we eat, excess kilojoules are converted into fat by our bodies and stored. So, to lose weight, we must eat fewer kilojoules than our bodies need, thereby forcing them to find energy by burning stored fat.

Proteins are an essential part of everyone's diet, regardless of age, because they build up and repair body tissues and produce biological substances such as some hormones and enzymes. They are especially important during periods when new tissue is formed, such as child growth, pregnancy and recovery from illness.

Food proteins differ in composition and, although we need all types to rebuild tissue, some foods are particularly good sources for body building and growth; for example, milk, meat, eggs, fish, nuts and soya beans. Proteins should make up 15 percent of our daily kilojoule allowance.

Carbohydrates include all starches and sugars. Sugars are found in foods such as sweets, honey, marmalade, jam, cakes, fruits and some vegetables. Starches occur in flour and all flour products, as well as in rice and in some vegetables; for example, potatoes and pumpkin. Unrefined starches – whole-grain cereals and breads made from whole-wheat flour, for example – add fibre to our diets as well as essential vitamins and minerals.

Carbohydrates should make up 55 percent of our daily kilojoule allowance.

Our bodies need *fats* to produce energy and for the absorption of fat-soluble vitamins. Foods rich in fats include butter, cream, oil and lard, as well as the fat in meat and oil in fish.

Fats should make up 30 percent of our daily kilojoule allowance.

Most foods contain at least some of the essential *minerals*, which our bodies need for vital processes. Iron, for instance, is needed for blood formation, and calcium for strong bones and teeth. Good sources of iron are liver, red meat, eggs and spinach; while an adequate supply of calcium is ensured by milk and dairy products, along with vitamin D. Other essential minerals are phosphorus, iodine, magnesium and potassium.

Vitamins, essential for health and wellbeing, may be either fat-soluble (vitamins A, E and D) or water-soluble (B-complex vitamins and vitamin C). Vitamin A is found in yellow vegetables such as carrots and pumpkin, yellow fruit and spinach; vitamin D is found in fish oils, margarine, and in sunlight; and nuts are a good source of vitamin E. Vitamin C is found in citrus fruits, guavas, tomatoes, potatoes, strawberries and broccoli. Some sources of B-complex vitamins are whole-grain foods and enriched cereals.

Energy requirements for healthy people are determined by their level of activity, gender, age and body build. People who are ill have different energy requirements.

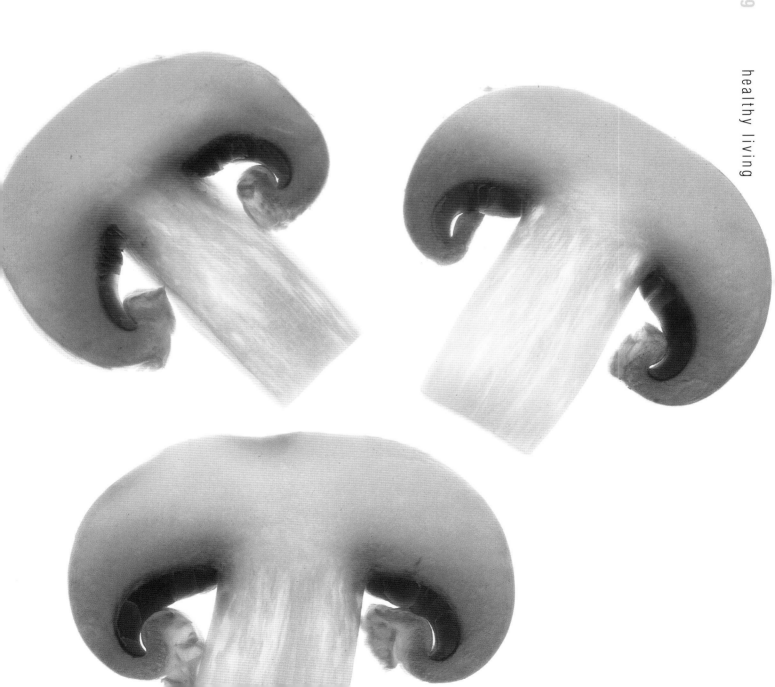

DIETARY GUIDELINES FOR HEALTHY PEOPLE
Daily nutritional requirements in terms of the food groups

FOODS	RECOMMENDED DAILY INTAKE	PORTION SIZES
Group 1 *Foods rich in* *calcium* milk, skimmed milk powder, yoghurt, buttermilk cheese, cream cheese, cottage cheese	children: 500 ml adults: 400 ml pregnant and lactating women: 650 ml 30 g	
Group 2 *Foods rich in* *protein* meat (lamb, beef, mutton, pork, venison etc.) eggs legumes, nuts	2 or more portions 1 (all ages) 2 or more portions	children up to 2: 30 g other children and adults: 90-110 g, cooked weight older children and adults: 30 g
Group 3 *Foods rich in* *vitamins and minerals* *Vitamin C* raw guavas, pawpaw, mango, citrus fruits, strawberries, pineapple, tomatoes, cabbage, broccoli, lettuce *Vitamin A* yellow peaches, apricots, pawpaw, mango, carrots, pumpkin, peas, green beans, avocado *Other vitamins* *and minerals* apples, bananas, peaches, grapes, potatoes, cauliflower onions, raisins, dried fruit, etc.	choose 4 portions in total choose *at least* 1 portion from this group choose *at least* 1 portion from this group 1 portion *after* choosing vitamin A and C sources	children up to 2: 30 g other children and adults: 1 fruit, 125 ml juice, or 100 g vegetables children up to 2: 30 g other children and adults: 1 fruit, 125 ml juice, or 100 g vegetables
Group 4 *Foods rich in* *carbohydrates,* *B-complex* *vitamins and minerals* bread, rusks cake, cereals, rice, noodles (select whole-grain types)	choose 4 or more portions	babies and children: choose portions according to their energy requirements Adults: 1 slice of bread or cake 100 g cereals, 100 g rice or noodles
Group 5 *Foods rich in fats* butter, margarine oil, cream	15 g or more of one of these sources	babies and children: choose portions according to their energy requirements

COMPILING HEALTHY MENUS

The most important point is to ensure that meals are *nutritionally balanced*. When planning menus, consult the Dietary guidelines for healthy people (page 10). Serve a fresh vegetable or fruit at least once, but preferably twice, a day. It's better to eat fruit, vegetables and whole-grain cereals as a source of carbohydrates rather than to eat too many sweets, cakes and puddings.

Take the following factors into account as well to ensure that meals look appetising and satisfy the taste buds:
- We experience food with all our senses, so an appealing *colour* combination of the different foods on the plate will help stimulate our appetites. Remember that the colours must complement one another. Garnishes such as fresh parsley and other herbs also add colour.
- Vary the *texture* of foods within one course; for example, croutons or parsley with soup. Vary the textures between courses as well; for example, alternate cooked food with a crisp salad, or serve a smooth dessert after a meal filled with raw and coarse-textured foods.
- Vary bland foods and those with a strong *flavour*, but don't have too many strong flavours at the same meal. Don't serve more than one kind of curry, for example, or more than one course with the same main ingredient; for example, tomato soup and tomato bredie.
- Don't serve too many foods prepared in the same way at one meal; for example, serve roast foods with a fresh salad and have stewed fruit for dessert.
- Alternate hot and cold courses.

SHOPPING FOR FOOD

HERE ARE SOME TIPS:
- PLAN YOUR MENU BEFOREHAND, MAKE A LIST OF WHAT TO BUY – AND STICK TO IT.
- KNOW THE PRICES OF FOODS YOU BUY REGULARLY, SO YOU CAN KEEP A CHECK ON COSTS.
- CHECK THE WEIGHT AND PRICE OF DIFFERENT BRANDS, SO YOU CAN BUY THE BEST VALUE.
- GET TO KNOW THE GRADING OF MEATS AND OTHER FOOD-STUFFS, AND BUY ACCORDING TO THE QUALITY YOU NEED.
- TAKE ADVANTAGE OF SPECIAL OFFERS, BUT BE PRACTICAL ABOUT IT.
- BUY VEGETABLES AND FRUITS IN SEASON, WHEN THEY'RE CHEAPER.

GLOSSARY

We often see and hear terms such as 'irradiation', 'additives' and 'antioxidants' mentioned in connection with nutrition and health, but it's seldom explained what they mean. Here are some definitions:

Additives are substances, not normally consumed as food by themselves, that are added to foods to give them certain characteristics, such as colour (e.g. tartrazine in margarine), flavour (e.g. flavour enhancers such as monosodium glutamate), texture (e.g. soya protein), a higher nutritional content (e.g. cereals fortified with iron, vitamins and/or minerals), or to guard against spoilage (commercially produced bread and herbs last longer because of the additives in them).

Alternative therapies are treatments other than allopathic or conventional medicine, and includes homeopathy, naturopathy, acupuncture, acupressure, herbal remedies, chiropractic, etc. If you're considering trying an alternative therapy, first find out how safe it is and how it may interact with conventional practices. Making healthy choices requires knowing what all the options are.

Antioxidants are used, for instance, to prevent rancidity of fats in food and they may be taken as supplements. Vitamins A, C and E are known antioxidants.

Irradiation means, in effect, to sterilise foods by exposing them to energy and energy waves, similar to ultraviolet light and microwaves. Irradiation is used on certain foods to improve safety. It kills harmful micro-organisms and insects on wheat, spices, tea, fresh and frozen beef, lamb, pork, poultry, fresh fruit and vegetables, and can also stop potatoes from sprouting and delay the ripening of fruit such as apples and pears.

Organic crops are crops grown and processed in accordance with strict regulations regarding the use of fertilisers, herbicides, insecticides, fungicides, preservatives and other chemical ingredients. Many consumers perceive organic crops as being more 'natural' and therefore healthier – and are willing to pay more for organically grown foods – but this is not necessarily true in all cases. Both organic and conventional methods have advantages and disadvantages.

Supplements are intended to rectify nutrient imbalances in our bodies and to keep us as healthy as possible. In this belief, many people are prepared to pay a small fortune in the hope of optimising their health. If we eat a healthy diet, most of us should get sufficient nutrients for our bodies to function at their best without having to take supplements. Some people, however, may suffer from marginal nutritional deficiencies and need to take supplements to supply this need:
- Strict vegetarians may need calcium, iron, zinc, vitamin B_{12} and vitamin D
- Pregnant and lactating women may need iron, calcium and folate
- People taking medication or who are on treatment which may interfere with their appetite or the absorption of nutrients
- People who have illnesses that obstruct nutrient absorption or increase the need for nutrients
- Women who bleed excessively during menstruation
- People who have had an operation or who have to be bedridden for a long time
- People who are on a very strict diet, low in kilojoules (energy).

Always check with your doctor which supplements you may need, and in what quantities. Don't be swayed by the belief that if one dose is good for you, a double dose is twice as good; in fact, oversupplementation can be dangerous. So make sure that you *always* stick to the recommended dosage.

Pregnancy and breast-feeding

How healthily you eat before and during pregnancy and breast-feeding affects not only your own health, but also the growth, development and health of your child, as a newborn and for some time afterwards. Good nutrition *before* pregnancy is essential both to conception and to the healthy development of the foetus, so if you're planning to start a family, make sure that you're eating a healthy, balanced diet.

SPECIAL NUTRIENT NEEDS DURING PREGNANCY

Your nutrient needs during pregnancy and breast-feeding are higher than at any other time in your adult life. The Dietary guidelines for healthy people (page 10) and the Daily nutritional requirements (page 10) apply equally if you're pregnant, but you will need an extra 1 260 kJ or so every day for the last six months of your pregnancy. You will need:

- 10 g extra protein a day, throughout your pregnancy.
- The vitamins required for rapid cell growth, i.e. folate and vitamin B_{12}. Folate plays an important role in preventing neural tube defects, such as spina bifida. In general terms, a balanced diet should take care of folate needs, but it is important that you take daily folate supplements of at least 400 micrograms for at least one month *before* conception (assuming your pregnancy is planned) and for the first three months of pregnancy. In fact, it would be a good idea for girls after puberty, and young women on birth control pills, to supplement on folate.
  Good sources of folate: Leafy green vegetables, legumes, liver, oranges and orange juice, whole-wheat products.
  Good sources of vitamin B12: Meat, fish, eggs, milk products.
- Vitamin D and calcium, important for building the bones and skeleton of the foetus.
  Good sources of vitamin D: Fish oils, margarine, sunlight.
  Good sources of calcium: Milk, skimmed milk powder, yoghurt, buttermilk, cheese, fruit such as citrus fruit, vegetables such as broccoli.
- Iron. Your iron needs shoot up during pregnancy. The developing foetus draws on its mother's iron stores to create its own stores – enough iron to last through the first four to six months of life. Pregnant women should take a daily supplement of 30 mg (milligrams) of iron during the last six months of pregnancy.
  Good sources of iron: Liver, oysters, red meat, fish, other meat such as chicken, dried fruit (especially raisins and prunes), legumes (cooked dried beans, peas, lentils), dark green vegetables, as well as vitamin C-rich foods such as oranges, guavas and tomatoes, which help improve iron absorption.

FOOD CRAVINGS AND AVERSIONS

PREGNANT WOMEN OFTEN HAVE CRAVINGS FOR – AND SOMETIMES AVERSIONS TO – CERTAIN FOODS AND DRINKS, AND SOMETIMES EVEN CRAVE THINGS SUCH AS CLAY, SAND AND STARCH (WHICH IS KNOWN AS 'PICA').

CONTRARY TO POPULAR BELIEF, HOWEVER, THESE DO NOT REFLECT A REAL PHYSIOLOGICAL NEED BUT MAY BE THE RESULT OF HORMONAL CHANGES, WHICH MAY INFLUENCE TASTE AND SMELL.

WEIGHT GAIN

Pregnant women, the saying goes, should eat for two, but this is one piece of advice that you should *not* follow! Weight gain, while a normal part of pregnancy, should be within these parameters:

Underweight women (BMI* of less than 19,8): 12,5–18 kg
Normal-weight women (BMI of 19,8–26): 11,5–16 kg
Overweight women (BMI of 26–29+): 7–11,5 kg
Women carrying twins: 16–20,5 kg
* BMI: An index that measures weight in relation to height, by dividing the weight (in kg) by the square of the height (in metres).

$$BMI = \frac{Weight\ (kg)}{Height\ (m)^2}$$

For example, a weight of 60 kg and a height of 1,64 metres will give a BMI of 26,8

Dieting is unadvisable for pregnant women; so if you've gained more than the expected amount of weight early in your pregnancy, do *not* try to diet during the last few weeks. And if you've suddenly gained a lot of weight, and retain a lot of fluid, do not consider it 'normal' – it could indicate the onset of hypertension (high blood pressure) and could lead to **pre-eclampsia** (see Glossary). Tell your doctor or midwife if you put on weight like this, so that they can take action if necessary.

EXERCISE DURING PREGNANCY

If you're active and physically fit, and your pregnancy is normal, you can continue exercising throughout your pregnancy, but you should adjust your exercise programme as needed. Ask your doctor for advice. Exercising regularly offers a number of advantages, which may include: stress relief, muscle toning, weight control, less back pain, easier labour, the prevention of gestational diabetes (page 51) and a faster recovery after childbirth.

A word of warning: Consult your doctor or clinic before starting, or continuing with, an exercise programme.

Here are some guidelines:

- Exercise regularly, at least three times a week.
- Stop if you feel overheated, especially in hot, humid weather.
- Drink enough fluids before, during and after exercising.
- Avoid jarring or jerky movements, or any activity that may cause abdominal trauma.
- Stop exercising if you experience discomfort; for instance, if your heart rate exceeds 140 beats a minute; if you are breathing too hard; or if you have a burning sensation in your lungs.
- Adjust your diet to your level of activity; if you're really active, for example, you can have more food.

SPECIAL PRECAUTIONS DURING PREGNANCY

When you're pregnant, you should strive to be as healthy as possible, for your own and your baby's sake. The following precautions are particularly important:

- Stop smoking. Both the expectant mother and the foetus are at risk if the mother smokes. Smoking restricts the blood supply to the growing foetus and so limits the amount of oxygen available; it also restricts the removal of wastes from the foetus. Cigarette smoking also increases the need for certain nutrients, such as vitamin C, and tends to increase the risk for a number of conditions, such as premature birth, spontaneous abortion and babies with a **low birth weight** (see Glossary).
- Stop taking alcohol and drugs. Certain substances can cross the placental barrier and affect the foetus negatively. A baby whose mother drank excessive amounts of alcohol during her pregnancy could become an addict, or suffer from Foetal Alcohol Syndrome, a group of symptoms including mental and physical retardation. Babies suffering from the syndrome often have facial and body deformities. Mothers who are drug users can pass their addiction on to their babies.
- Be careful when taking medicines. Pregnant women should ask their doctor or pharmacist for advice if they're taking medicines, to make sure that what they take is safe for their own, and their unborn baby's, health. Many medicinal products carry a warning for pregnant or breast-feeding women.

NOTE: Viruses such as rubella, which can cause German measles and other conditions, may also be transferred from the mother to the foetus, especially during the vulnerable first few months, when most of the unborn child's development takes place. This could result in a congenital abnormality in your baby.

PROBLEMS DURING PREGNANCY

Expectant mothers often experience one or more of the following problems:

Morning sickness, which can be as mild as feeling faintly queasy or as serious as extreme nausea and vomiting. If it is excessive, vomiting can be a risk to maintaining the electrolyte (sodium and water) balance in your body, and may necessitate a few days in hospital until the balance is regained.

It's thought that morning sickness may be the result of hormonal changes occurring in pregnant women, especially during the first three months.

Here are some tips for combating morning sickness:

- Get up slowly when you arise in the morning, so you won't feel nauseous.
- Eat crackers or dry toast before getting up, which helps relieve feelings of queasiness.
- Eat small meals, often (you could get nauseous if you're too full).

- Don't drink with your meals, for the same reason.
- Avoid foods whose smell triggers nausea (many women find that smells, particularly cooking smells, bring on the symptoms).
- If you're taking vitamin and mineral supplements, do so after you've eaten to avoid nausea, or at a time of day when the nausea is at its lowest.
- Chewing gum or sucking hard sweets settles your stomach.
- Try to eat when you're not feeling nauseous, so that you can be sure you will take in the nutrients you need.

Heartburn is common during pregnancy. The growing foetus puts more and more pressure on your stomach, which can cause stomach acids to back up and create a burning sensation in your throat. If you're going to take antacids, make sure that they're safe and use them in moderation.

Here are some tips for relieving heartburn:

- Eat small meals, often; if you're too full, gastric acids can push up into your throat.
- Avoid wearing clothes that are tight around the breasts and abdomen, because the constriction has the same effect.
- Drink liquids between meals, not with your meals, and sip them slowly, for the same reason.
- For the same reason, eat slowly and chew your food well.
- Sit up to eat meals, and wait at least an hour before lying down to take a rest.
- Avoid spicy and greasy foods, as well as caffeine and alcohol, which may make the problem worse.
- Don't exercise directly after eating; if you're too full, heartburn could result.

Constipation: Pregnancy hormones alter the muscle tone of the digestive tract and the growing baby puts increasing pressure on your organs. A diet high in fibre, drinking plenty of water and exercising will help. Take laxatives only if they are prescribed by your doctor, and avoid mineral oils such as liquid paraffin because they affect the absorption of fat-soluble vitamins A, D and E.

Hypertension (high blood pressure) may be a pre-existing condition, or it may develop during pregnancy. Watch it very carefully, as it can lead to pre-eclampsia, a condition which affects almost all the mother's organs. If it progresses, convulsions, called **eclampsia** (see Glossary), may result. This is very serious and a cause for great concern. Treatment for pre-eclampsia concentrates on regulating blood pressure levels and preventing convulsions.

BREAST-FEEDING

Breast-feeding your baby has many advantages: the milk is available in the right strength and concentration; the chances of contaminated water being used to clean bottle teats are eliminated; and, most importantly, your baby is protected against disease as several protective substances are secreted in breast milk.

When you're lactating and breast-feeding, you produce about 750 ml of milk a day. You need extra energy to produce breast milk, so your daily kilojoule intake should be increased by about 2 000 kJ a day. For example, if your normal energy intake is about 5 600 kJ a day, during breast-feeding it should be about 7 600 kJ.

It's commonly believed that drinking lots of fluid while breast-feeding will help you produce more milk, but this is not so. You should, however, drink at least 1 litre of fluid daily to protect against dehydration. Water is better than soft drinks or fruit juice if you want to lose weight as well.

Taking supplements while you're breast-feeding shouldn't be necessary, unless your diet is inadequate, or you're a teenager, or if you have a special health problem, where you need extra supplements.

Because breast-feeding uses up kilojoules, the period while you're lactating and breast-feeding your baby is the best time for you to lose the extra weight you put on during pregnancy. Concentrate on low-fat, high-fibre foods and continue with, or step up, your exercise programme.

A few precautions while you're breast-feeding:

- Don't eat too many strongly flavoured or spicy foods. They may alter the taste of breast milk, and your baby may refuse to drink.
- Avoid alcohol, as even a small quantity enters breast milk very easily.
- Reduce your intake of coffee, cola drinks and some sports drinks, as the caffeine they contain may cause irritability and wakefulness in your baby.

- As a precaution, always consult your doctor before taking medicines to make sure they're safe, as medications and drugs are also secreted in breast milk.
- Ask your doctor's advice about taking oral contraceptives. They contain estrogen, which reduces both the volume and the protein content of breast milk.

Remember that breast-feeding mothers who are drug or alcohol addicts can cause their babies to become addicts too, because their babies get the substances through breast milk.

FEEDING YOUR BABY

Breast milk is the perfect food for the young infant; with the exception of vitamin D, it provides all the nutrients a healthy infant needs for the first four to six months of its life. There are instances, however, where a mother cannot breast-feed and will have to give her baby formula for six months to a year, then change to cow's milk (provided that her baby is not allergic to it). Ask your doctor or dietician for advice.

Many kinds of formula are available commercially: some consist of cow's milk treated to simulate breast milk; others are made from soya milk for babies who are allergic to cow's milk. Premature babies need special formulas.

Here are some guidelines:
- Clean bottles and teats properly. Sterilise them for a young baby.
- Use slightly cooled boiled water to mix the formula.
- Dentists advise against putting an infant to bed with a bottle, as the milk that remains in the mouth could cause tooth decay.
- Toddlers one to two years of age should be given full-fat milk, not low-fat or fat-free milk.
- Your baby also needs to drink water, one of the most important nutrients for an infant; if he or she has a fever or diarrhoea, it's easy to become dehydrated, in a very short time, and this may be life-threatening.

WHEN TO INTRODUCE SOLID FOODS

Introduce solid foods gradually. You can start as early as four to six months – which is when the ability to swallow solid food develops – provided that your baby can sit up (with support) and can control his or her head movements. The following are important:

- Your baby's nutrient needs (iron and vitamin C are required first)
- Physical readiness to handle different forms of food
- Possible allergic reactions: introduce new foods one at a time so that you can eliminate any that seem to cause a reaction.

Commercially prepared baby foods are of good quality and perfectly safe, but you can also cook vegetables and meat yourself and mash or grind them. Take care when adding salt, however, as an infant's kidneys cannot cope with sodium (salt), and salty foods may cause problems.

This table gives you some idea of when to introduce various solid foods:

AGE (months)	FOODS
4–6	Iron-fortified rice cereal, followed by other single-grain cereals, mixed with breast milk, formula or water puréed vegetables and fruits, one by one (perhaps vegetables before fruits, so baby will learn to like their less sweet flavours)
6–8	Infant breads and crackers mashed vegetables and fruits and their juices
8–10	Foods from the table finely cut meats, fish, chicken; casseroles, cheese, yoghurt, tofu, eggs and legumes
10–12	Continue to introduce a variety of nutritious foods

Six months of age is also a good time to start teaching your baby to drink from a cup, and at eight months to a year, she or he will be able to sit up and handle finger foods.

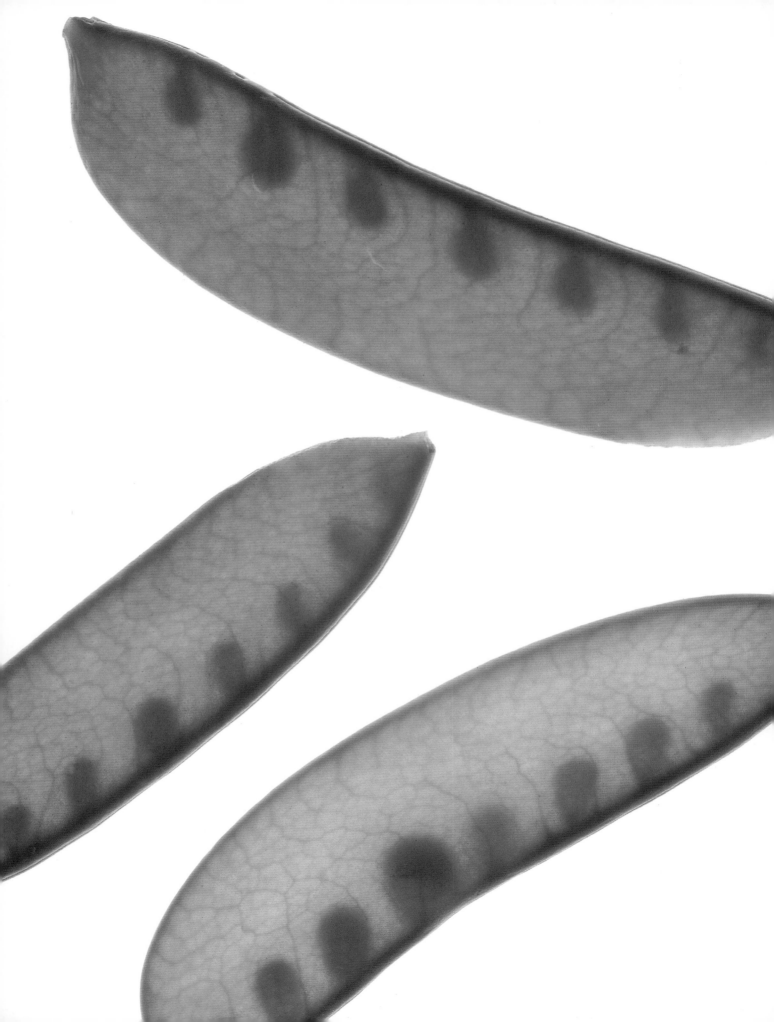

GLOSSARY

Amniotic sac: The 'water bag' in the uterus, in which the foetus floats.

Eclampsia: A toxic condition of unknown cause that sometimes develops in the last three months of pregnancy, and is characterised by high blood pressure, abnormal weight gain and convulsions.

Embryo: The developing baby from conception to eight weeks after conception.

Foetus: The developing baby from eight weeks after conception until birth.

Low birth weight: Normal birth weight for a full-term baby is 3 000 to 4 000 g (3 to 4 kg). A birth weight of less than 2 500 g (2,5 kg) probably indicates poor health in the newborn, and poor nutritional status of the mother during pregnancy.

Placenta: An organ that develops inside the uterus early in pregnancy. In the placenta, the blood of the mother and the unborn baby circulate in close proximity and exchange materials: the foetus receives nutrients and oxygen via the placenta, while the mother's blood picks up carbon dioxide and other waste materials from the foetus, to be excreted via her lungs and kidneys.

Pre-eclampsia: A toxic condition of pregnancy characterised by high blood pressure, protein in the urine, abnormal weight gain, and oedema (fluid retention).

Umbilical cord: The rope-like structure through which the foetus's veins and arteries reach the placenta. The umbilical cord is also the route of nourishment and oxygen into the foetus, and the route of waste disposal from it.

Uterus or womb: The muscular organ in which the infant develops before birth.

Toddlers and young children

Among the many worries parents have about a young child is his or her appetite.

Up to the age of about one year there's no problem as an infant's appetite is robust because he or she is growing so fast. By five months of age, for example, an infant's weight is double that at birth and by the age of a year, the weight has trebled. How well an infant grows *directly* reflects his or her nutritional wellbeing.

At about one year of age, a healthy child's appetite usually slows down, but this is perfectly normal. A young child's appetite fluctuates, as well as his or her taste for certain foods. What parents should remember is that each child's growth rate is different; what is important is that their child's weight should fall within a *broad* spectrum of the normal height and weight for their age. Ask your doctor or the clinic for a growth chart to use as a guide.

Parents do, however, need to teach their children to choose the right foods and to encourage healthy play and exercise. If their child is overweight, they may find that this is because he or she is eating in response to outside stimuli such as TV commercials, ignoring the body's inbuilt appetite-regulating signals.

DEVELOPING HEALTHY EATING HABITS

In order to provide all the nutrients a growing child needs, meals and snacks should include a variety of foods from each food group (see Dietary guidelines for healthy people, page 10). Steady growth during childhood requires a gradual increase in the intake of most nutrients, and children should, ideally, store nutrients before adolescence, when there is a major growth spurt. Calcium, in particular, is important – the denser their bones, the better prepared children will be for growth spurts.

Developing healthy eating habits in a child is essential. The great challenge is to give children nutritious meals and snacks *they will enjoy*, and to instil in them a desire to choose such foods. Overweight children, especially, need to be persuaded to eat nutrient-dense foods (which contain plenty of nutrients without too much fat), such as skimmed milk, low-fat yoghurt, fruit and vegetables (prepared without sugar or fat), that will meet all their energy requirements and also help them to lose weight – or at least not put on more kilograms! Active children who are a normal weight, as well as underweight children, may have foods higher in kilojoules, such as ice cream and sweets, but these should form part of their healthy eating plan, and not be extras.

How you go about developing healthy eating habits in your child has a number of important aspects: their food preferences, their attitude to foods, and strong ideas about when and what they eat.

Food preferences: As a general guide, children seem to prefer:

- Raw vegetables, cut into fingers, rather than cooked vegetables
- Mild-tasting food (especially younger children)

- Smooth food, without lumps
- Foods piled separately on the plate, rather than mixed together
- Foods that look appealing – create interest with a variety of shapes and colours, and avoid any hard, round shapes, on which your child could choke.

Most young children like to sit at small tables when they eat, and prefer easy-to-use eating utensils.

Power struggles: Negative feelings about food often start at an early age. Children of two or three start to assert their independence, and power struggles will ensue if parents, in an attempt to do what they think is best, try to control every aspect of their child's eating. This sets a pattern of resistance that may grow worse as the child gets older. Remember: parents are responsible for *what* a child eats; a child is responsible for *how much* (or even whether) he or she eats.

Introducing new foods: Introduce new foods one at a time, in small quantities. The best time is at the start of the meal, when your child is hungry. Ignore it if he or she refuses to eat the new food and simply have it available again at the next meal.

Mealtimes: The ideal scenario would be for meals to follow playtimes, otherwise your child will be in a hurry to finish eating so that he or she can go out and play. Meals should be served at the table, not in front of the TV, otherwise TV programmes soon become the determining factor for mealtimes. Children who eat while they're watching TV tend to become obese, because they are inactive and also because they're tempted by the fast foods they see advertised.

Snacks: A child's idea of a snack is more likely to be a chocolate or a couple of crisps than fruit or unflavoured yoghurt. Your best course of action to introduce nutritious snacks is to include them in your child's healthy eating plan, so that he or she will not consider them to be 'forbidden' foods. Offer your children pieces of cheese, sausages, small sandwiches cut into animal shapes, pieces of fruit, vegetable sticks and so on.

Role models: Children tend to copy adults, even if their elders are unaware of it. They also watch what other children eat, as well as their teachers and other people with whom they come into contact. If the role model eats healthily it's a plus; if he or she doesn't, it can cause a problem with your child. Don't discourage your child from eating what other people eat as this will make the food forbidden and therefore desirable; rather try to instil good habits by positive example.

Nutrition and the aged

The effects of nutrition and environment on longevity have provided incentives for researchers to keep on asking questions about how and why human beings age. Healthy habits, such as following a healthy diet and taking exercise, seem to have an influence on people's health and therefore on their physiological age; good nutrition and disease prevention are other important issues.

THE RELATIONSHIP BETWEEN NUTRITION AND DISEASE

There is a strong relationship between good nutrition and disease prevention:
- A healthy energy (kilojoule) intake (see Dietary guidelines for healthy people, page 10) helps prevent obesity, diabetes mellitus and cardiovascular diseases such as atherosclerosis and hypertension. It may also guard against certain forms of cancer, such as colon cancer.
- An adequate intake of essential nutrients (see Dietary guidelines for healthy people, page 10) prevents deficiency diseases.
- A varied, balanced diet (see Healthy eating for older adults, page 19) may protect against certain types of cancer, such as colon cancer, especially if it includes fruit and vegetables and plenty of fibre.
- Calcium helps protect against osteoporosis (see page 19).

ENERGY NEEDS

Our energy needs decline the older we get; as a general rule, an estimated 5 percent per decade. One of the reasons for this is that as we get older, we also reduce our level of physical activity. As a consequence, lean body mass (our muscles) diminishes and our metabolic rate slows down.

Many older people cut down on foods/nutrients for these reasons, which can have quite dramatic effects,

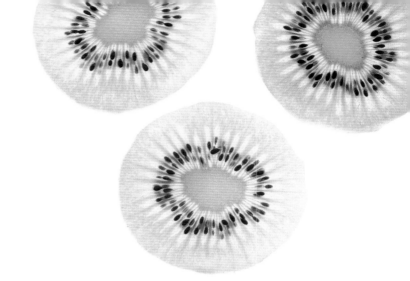

especially when it comes to a reduced intake of water, energy (kilojoules), fibre-rich foods, protein, vitamins A and D, iron, zinc and calcium. The following are the effects of ageing on these substances, along with comments on the effects and, in some instances, what should be done to alleviate them:

Water

Effect of ageing: Lack of thirst and decreased total body water make dehydration likely.

Comments: Mild dehydration is a common cause of confusion. Difficulty obtaining water or getting to the bathroom may compound the problem.

Energy (kilojoules)

Effect of ageing: Energy needs decrease.

Comments: Physical activity will slow down the decline.

Fibre

Effects of ageing: Likelihood of constipation increases with a low intake, as do changes in the gastrointestinal tract.

Comments: Inadequate water intake and lack of physical activity, along with some medications, compound the problem. Try to increase the quantity of fibre-rich foods eaten.

Protein

Effects of ageing: Energy needs decrease.

Comments: Increase the intake of low-fat, high-fibre legumes and grains that meet protein and other nutrient needs.

Vitamin A

Effects of ageing: Absorption rate may increase. Vitamin A is an antioxidant and very important for older people.

Comments: RDA (recommended daily allowance, may be high.

Vitamin D

Effects of ageing: Increased likelihood of inadequate intake; skin synthesis declines.

Comments: Limited daily exposure to sunlight may be of benefit.

Iron

Effects of ageing: In women, status improves after menopause; deficiencies are linked to chronic blood losses, as during menstruation, and low stomach acid output.

Comments: Adequate stomach acid is required for the absorption of iron. Antacids or other medicine may aggravate an iron deficiency. Vitamin C and meat increase the absorption rate.

Zinc

Effects of ageing: Intakes may be low and absorption rate reduced, but needs may also decrease.

Comments: Medication interferes with absorption; a deficiency may supress the appetite and sense of taste. To increase the intake of zinc, eat meat, fish, and poultry.

Calcium

Effects of ageing: Intakes may be low; osteoporosis common.

Comments: Stomach discomfort commonly limits milk intake; calcium substitutes, i.e. foods made with milk, are needed.

HEALTHY EATING FOR OLDER ADULTS

A healthy daily eating plan for older adults would include:

- 2-3 servings (60 g each) of lean meat, poultry, fish, eggs, dried beans or peas, nuts
- 2-3 servings (250 ml [1 cup] each) of milk, cheese or yoghurt
- 6 or more servings of whole-grain breads or cereals
- 2-4 servings (125 ml [½ cup] each) fruit
- 3-5 servings (125 ml [½ cup] each) vegetables

OSTEOPOROSIS

The term literally means porous bones and indicates reduced bone density. People who suffer from osteoporosis run a high risk of fractures, often of the upper thigh and hip, which necessitates hip-replacement surgery.

There are several causes of osteoporosis, both hereditary and environmental, and the onset of the disease doesn't necessarily start when we're older. Loss of bone density can start in young people who have any of the risk factors given below, and it will get worse with age.

RISK FACTORS FOR DEVELOPING OSTEOPOROSIS

A number of risk factors have been identified for developing osteoporosis, and these may have a high or a moderate correlation. Other risk factors, although not yet proved, may also have an effect.

High-correlation risk factors for osteoporosis include: Being a woman (especially being blonde and fair-skinned), being thin, being postmenopausal, advanced age, alcohol abuse, anorexia nervosa, chronic steroid use, rheumatoid arthritis, having had ovaries surgically removed.

Protective factors include being black-skinned, and long-term use of estrogens.

Moderate-correlation risk factors for osteoporosis include: Chronic thyroid hormone use, cigarette smoking, diabetes (Type 1), early menopause, excessive antacid use, a low-calcium diet, sedentary lifestyle or immobility, vitamin D deficiency.

Protective factors include having given birth, and having a normal body weight.

Unproven but probably important risk factors include: Caffeine use, a family history of osteoporosis, a high-fibre, high-protein, or high-sodium diet.

Protective factors include a high-calcium diet and regular physical activity.

COMBATING OSTEOPOROSIS

Following a nutritionally sound eating plan, high in calcium and vitamin D, is absolutely essential. Our bones are denser if we're active rather than sedentary, which means that physical exercise plays an equally important role. Muscle strength and bone strength go together, and weight-bearing physical activity, such as walking, running or dancing, will stimulate our bones to deposit minerals. The more dietary calcium our bodies retain, the greater the bone density and, potentially, the lower the risk of developing osteoporosis.

The following are the recommended daily calcium requirements for:

adolescents	1 300 mg
adults	1 000 mg
adults over 50 years	1 200 mg

Food sources of calcium are: Milk and milk products such as cheese and yoghurt, broccoli, and calcium-fortified products, such as milk drinks and calcium supplements.

If you don't drink milk, for whatever reason, it's more difficult to increase your intake of calcium. Here are some tips for increasing your calcium intake without drinking milk:

- Use milk or powdered milk to make puddings and custards.
- Vegetarians or those allergic to milk may use calcium-fortified soya milk or tofu.
- Eat soft-boned fish, such as salmon, as well as canned fish, including the soft bones.

ARTHRITIS

The most common type of arthritis, that disables older people in particular, is *osteoarthritis*, a painful swelling of the joints. There are many so-called remedies for arthritis, but researchers maintain that no known diet or remedy prevents, or cures, the condition. Depending on the individual, certain foods sometimes make the pain worse, and it's been shown that being overweight also plays a role. If you lose weight, it will relieve the pain and make exercising easier.

Rheumatoid arthritis, a disease of the immune system, is characterised by painful inflammation of the joints, the soft tissues around joints, the ligaments and cartilage. The immune system depends on good nutrition, so if your daily eating plan lacks some nutrients, you may find that your arthritis becomes worse. Some sufferers find that foods such as milk and milk products may stimulate the immune system to attack and make the pain worse. In this case, limit intake of milk and milk products but make sure that you take calcium supplements.

Some research shows that the eating plan recommended for heart health – one low in saturated fats and high in omega-3 fatty acids – may help prevent or relieve the inflammation in the joints that makes both types of arthritis so painful. (See page 42 for more information.

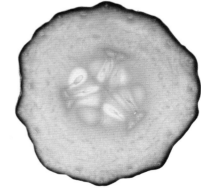

Sports nutrition

Active people need a diet packed with **nutrient-dense foods** (see Glossary). A daily eating plan high in carbohydrates (60 percent or more of total kilojoules), low in fat (25 percent of total kilojoules) and adequate in protein (12–15 percent of total kilojoules) will ensure that glycogen and other nutrient stores are kept full. This type of eating plan will help to control weight, provide enough fibre, and supply all other nutrients as well.

If you're training intensively, your energy requirements may outstrip your capacity to eat enough foods to obtain the nutrients you need to meet these requirements, and you may need extra carbohydrates and fats.

Physically active people also need protein, though the quantities and kinds are often heatedly debated; meat and milk products, for instance, are rich sources of protein, but they're also high in saturated fats. If you choose a wide variety of protein sources, and include legumes, grains and vegetables in your eating plan, you will also get the carbohydrates needed for your body to provide energy.

EATING BEFORE EXERCISE

Although many sportsmen and -women believe a particular food is essential to enhance performance, no single food has been shown to improve speed, skill or strength in competitive events.

As a sensible pre-exercise regimen, you should eat a meal three to five hours before competition to allow your stomach time to empty before you start (fibre in the digestive tract attracts water from the blood and causes stomach problems during exercise). This meal should include plenty of fluids, be light and easy to digest, and be made up primarily of carbohydrate-rich foods. Good choices are breads, potatoes, pasta and fruit juices; you can also make a liquid meal that's easy to digest, such as fat-free milk or fruit juice and fruit mixed in a blender.

EATING AFTER EXERCISE

Carbohydrate-containing drinks are usually the first type of food consumed after a competitive event. Choose nutrient-dense foods such as low-fat milk or low-fat foods (because they're light and easy to digest) and avoid foods high in fats and protein for the first few hours after vigorous exercise. Once your body's carbohydrate stores have been replenished and you start to feel hungry, you can eat other foods.

HYDRATION AND DEHYDRATION

It's important to ensure your body doesn't become dehydrated while you're exercising and that the electrolyte level and your body's water balance are maintained. Endurance athletes, for instance, can easily lose 1,5 litres or more of fluid during each hour of activity, so they, and other sportsmen and women, should hydrate before they start, and replace fluid losses during and after exercise. The following hydration schedule will help you:

When to drink	Quantity of fluid
2 hours before exercise	750 ml (3 cups)
10–15 minutes before	500 ml (2 cups)
every 15 minutes	
during exercise	250 ml (1 cup)
after exercise	500 ml (2 cups)

Ordinary cool water is recommended for noncompetitive active people, as it leaves the digestive tract rapidly to enter the tissues, and cools the body from the inside. For professional endurance athletes, however, sport drinks may be better, as they will supplement the body's stores of glycogen, which is needed for energy.

REPLACING WATER

Water is the crucial nutrient for all of us, but especially for those taking part in physical activities. Our bodies lose water through perspiration and breathing (exhaled as water vapour) and we could become dehydrated. The first symptom of dehydration is fatigue; a water loss of 1–2 percent of body weight can affect performance and if the water loss is about 7 percent of body weight, you could collapse.

Our bodies cool themselves by perspiring. In hot, humid weather perspiration doesn't evaporate well because the surrounding air is already high in water content. If perspiration doesn't evaporate, little cooling takes place and heatstroke – which can be fatal – may result.

To reduce the risk of heatstroke, drink enough fluid before and during exercise (see hydration schedule above), rest in the shade if you're tired and wear lightweight clothing that allows perspiration to evaporate. Don't wear the rubber or plastic suits that supposedly promote weight loss during exercise – they *do* promote heavy perspiration but they also prevent evaporation, which can lead to heatstroke.

The symptoms of heatstroke are: Headache, nausea, dizziness, clumsiness and stumbling, excessive or very little perspiration, confusion or disorientation.

Hyperthermia (above-normal body temperature) and hypothermia (low body temperature) are equally dangerous. Inexperienced skiers or slow runners, for instance, who produce little body heat, may experience hypothermia, and so may swimmers. Even in cold weather our bodies still perspire and need fluid replacement, so it's important *always* to follow the hydration schedule when you're going to exercise.

REPLACING ELECTROLYTES

Usually, a well-balanced diet will see to it that the salts called **electrolytes** (see Glossary) are replenished in your body, but if you perspire a lot during exercise – such as when it's hot and humid, the exercise is vigorous, and your fitness level isn't quite up to scratch – it may be necessary for you to make sure yourself that the electrolytes are replenished.

If you lose electrolytes, you also lose water and this leads to dehydration. If you lose 2,5–5 kg or more a day from perspiring for several consecutive days, ordinary water may not be enough and you should take a sports drink, or a mixture of 2 ml (½ tsp) salt in 250 ml (1 cup) fruit juice, stirred into 1 litre (4 cups) water. Some sportsmen and -women take salt tablets to replace the electrolytes they lose through perspiration, but this isn't a good idea, as the tablets can irritate your stomach and cause vomiting, which will make the situation worse.

GLOSSARY

Electrolytes are salts that dissolve in water, and play a major role in maintaining the water balance in the body.

Nutrient-dense foods provide a maximum of nutrients, including carbohydrates, protein, fats, minerals and vitamins, for the amount of energy (kJ) they provide.

Food allergies

Certain foods and products, harmless and nutritious in themselves, may be enjoyed happily by many people but pose allergy problems for others. The reasons for allergic reactions aren't always properly understood, and continuing research seeks to unravel the mysteries.

ALLERGIES

The immune system acts as a defence mechanism, protecting our bodies from harmful substances such as bacteria and viruses and in so doing prevents illness. In the allergic (or atopic) person, there is a breakdown in the immune system, causing the body to react to a certain substance that is normally harmless. The atopic person may be sensitive to several **allergens** (see Glossary).

Allergies appear to have a genetic link, so a family history of eczema, for instance, may be present in parents and also appear in the children.

AN ALLERGIC REACTION

When a susceptible person comes into contact with an allergen, **antibodies** (see Glossary) called IgE (immunoglobulin E) immediately start working – in conjunction with special 'mast' cells in our bodies which release further substances, such as histamine – to attack the invading material. The result is an allergic reaction (see **food allergy** in the Glossary), with all its symptoms.

The site of the mast cells is also the site of the reaction; for example, the skin, nose, lungs or intestines. Depending on the site, the reaction may be vomiting and diarrhoea, hay fever, asthma, a blocked or runny nose, urticaria (hives) or eczema.

All kinds of substances may trigger an allergic reaction in susceptible people: pollen, pets' fur, dust mites, rubber, insect stings, fish and shellfish, milk and peanuts may all be potential allergens. Each allergy has classic symptoms; for example, violent sneezing in hay fever, but the symptoms are not exclusive to one type of allergy. That's why it's so difficult to know precisely which allergen is responsible, and this is why

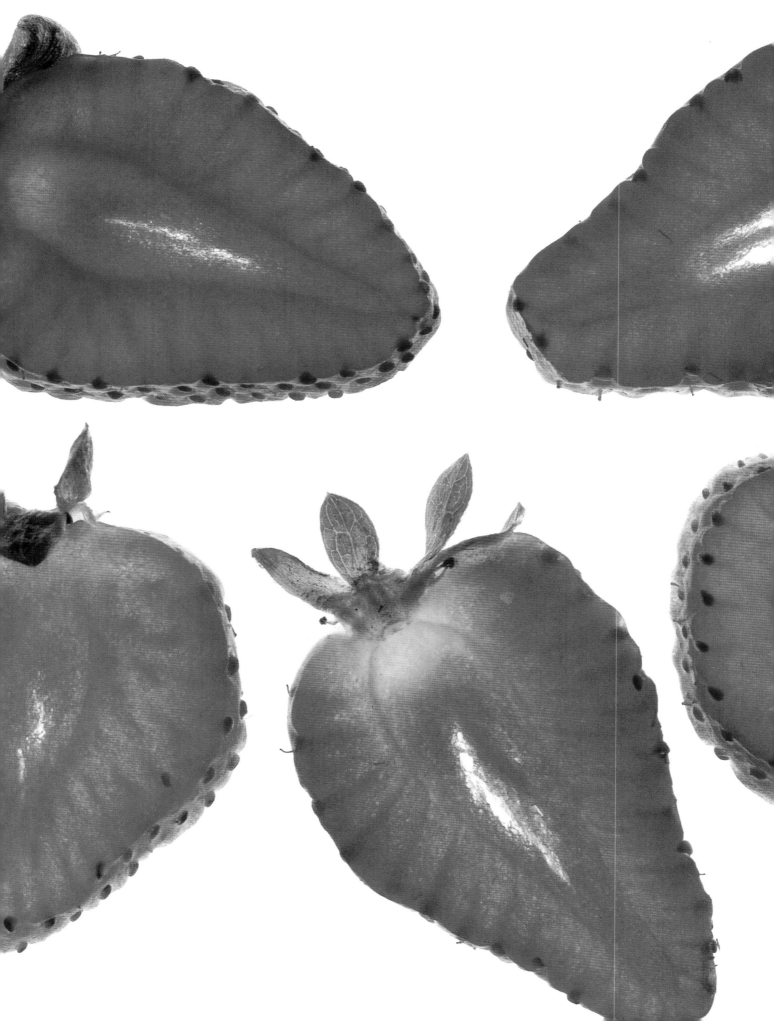

we should seek medical advice to find out what the allergen is, so that appropriate measures can be taken.

FOOD INTOLERANCE
(see Glossary)

Food intolerance is a broad term used to describe many negative symptoms associated with food intake, and includes any abnormal reaction that occurs as a result of eating the offending food. It's important to find out which food or foods are causing the problem, so that treatment may be prescribed. In some cases this may mean temporarily or permanently cutting down on the quantity of that food eaten; in others it may mean avoiding the offending food altogether.

Foods that most often cause adverse reactions include eggs, fish, shellfish, wheat and **gluten** (see Glossary), milk (lactose intolerance), peanuts and soya beans.

Adverse reactions may be caused by other factors, such as:

- MSG (monosodium glutamate).
- Certain chemicals in foods; for example, the natural laxative in prunes.
- Symptoms of ulcers or hernias becoming worse.
- Enzyme deficiencies, such as lactose intolerance, that cause symptoms difficult to distinguish from those of food allergies.
- Psychological reactions based on a belief that certain foods cause certain symptoms.

LACTOSE INTOLERANCE AND ALLERGY TO MILK

Lactose intolerance is a very common condition, which occurs because our bodies lack, or produce too little of, an enzyme called lactase. This enzyme's function is to break down lactose (milk sugar) into the simpler sugars, glucose and galactose, which are then absorbed by our bodies. If this doesn't happen, the undigested lactose passes to the colon where it causes irritation and the typical symptoms: bloating, pain, diarrhoea and flatulence. Temporary lactose intolerance can also be triggered by gastroenteritis, mainly in children.

The degree of intolerance varies from mild to quite severe. Some people, for instance, can eat yoghurt and some cheeses, but not drink milk.

When cow's milk is introduced to previously breast-fed babies, unpleasant symptoms related to dairy intolerance may arise because the baby's digestive system cannot cope with the different composition of cow's milk. For this reason, it's recommended that unmodified cow's milk should not be given before a child is six months old; in fact, some evidence suggests that breast-feeding for at least three months but preferably for four to six months may offer some protection against intolerance to cow's milk.

An allergy to milk, on the other hand, is relatively uncommon. It's usually restricted to young children, who generally outgrow the problem by the age of two or three. Classic symptoms include eczema, asthma, allergic rhinitis (constantly running nose), vomiting and diarrhoea.

COMBATING LACTOSE INTOLERANCE

Some foods that cause problems are more easily avoided than others; for example, strawberries or shellfish. Others, like dairy foods or wheat, are used in so many dishes and combinations that it makes avoidance much more difficult.

The most effective way to handle lactose intolerance is to follow a dairy-free diet. Great care must be taken, however, to ensure that the important nutrients in dairy products – such as protein, calcium, vitamins A, D and B_2 (riboflavin) – are obtained from other foods.

THE DAIRY-FREE DIET

Use the following guidelines to find out which foods you should avoid and which you should eat if you have a lactose intolerance:

Dairy products

Avoid these foods: Milk, evaporated milk, crème fraîche, fromage frais, quark, butter, buttermilk, cheese, cottage cheese, yoghurt

Use instead: Dairy substitutes such as soya 'milk', nut 'milk', rice 'milk' and tofu (soya bean curd)

Breads, cereals and baked goods

Avoid these foods: Foods containing dairy products, muesli and instant oats containing milk powder, cereal and energy bars, milk chocolate, fudge, toffee, cakes (unless they're stated to be milk- or lactose-free), Yorkshire pudding

Use instead: Arrowroot, bagels, pitta breads, pizza bases (but check the labels), meringues, good-quality dark chocolate, phyllo pastry (brush with oil), water biscuits, rice cakes, matzos, cream crackers, most plain breakfast cereals, All-Bran, Weetbix, cornflakes, rice, couscous, semolina, bulgur wheat, taco shells, poppadoms, tortilla chips, samoosas, rotis

Desserts and drinks

Avoid these foods: Coffee whitener, malted milk drinks, milk shakes, instant chocolate drinks, some instant coffees, custard, ice cream and some sorbets, pudding and batter mixes, chocolate, lemon curd

Use instead: Jellies, marshmallows, carob, mints, plain hard sweets, fruit ice lollies, sorbet

Fats and spreads

Avoid these foods: Dairy spreads, soft and hard margarine

Use instead: Vegetable oil, olive oil, kosher margarine, lard, vegetable fat, French dressing, mayonnaise

Sauces and condiments

Avoid these foods: Some prepared mustards, instant sauces, creamed pasta dishes, some instant gravies, some artificial sweeteners

Use instead: Relishes, chutney, pickles, soy sauce, vinegar, mustard powder, herbs and spices, most tomato-based pasta sauces, bouillon cubes, pesto, tomato sauce

Soups

Avoid these foods: Creamed soups

Use instead: French onion soup, bouillon and clear soups

Fruit

Avoid these foods: Canned and dried fruit with added lactose

Use instead: Fresh, canned and dried fruit without added lactose

Vegetables

Avoid these foods: Creamed vegetables, instant mashed potatoes

Use instead: Fresh, canned, dried and frozen vegetables (except creamed ones)

Meat, poultry and fish

Avoid these foods: Frankfurters and sausages containing dairy derivatives (see Notes below), ready-prepared creamed dishes, some battered and crumbed products

Use instead: Fresh or frozen poultry, fish and shellfish, canned tuna and salmon, canned meat (without sauces), sausages and burgers (but check the labels)

egetarian products

All vegan products may be used, as well as most other vegetable dishes, vegetarian 'sausages' and 'burgers'.

Notes

- Many dairy products and their derivatives are used in a wide range of processed foods. Check the ingredients list on product labels and avoid those containing: casein, caseinates, ghee, hydrolised casein, lactose, lactalbumin, milk sugar, milk solids, nonfat milk solids, skimmed milk whey, skimmed milk powder, hydrolised milk protein, whey, whey protein, whey sugar, and whey syrup sweetener.

- Ask the customer information service at your supermarket for information on products that are free of milk and their derivatives. Check the kosher shelves in larger stores for information too.

- Goat's and sheep's milk are often recommended as an alternative to cow's milk, but both contain lactose and will probably only be suitable for people with a *mild* lactose intolerance. The same applies to cheese and yoghurt made from these milks.

- Yoghurt is a fermented milk product that may contain bacteria that will change lactose to lactic acid. People with a mild lactose intolerance may therefore be able to eat yoghurt.

- You may find that sterilised UHT and evaporated milk may be tolerated in small quantities.

- Hard cheeses such as Parmesan and Cheddar are relatively low in lactose, so small quantities may be safe to eat. Experiment with the different kinds of cheeses to find out which you can tolerate.

- Soya 'milk' drinks are lactose-free, cholesterol-free, high in protein and sometimes fortified with calcium. Soya milk can be used as a substitute for milk in many dishes.

- Tofu is a high-protein, low-fat food made from soya beans. It can have a firm or soft texture and is available at most large supermarkets. It may also be UHT-treated.

WHEAT AND GLUTEN ALLERGY AND INTOLERANCE

Coeliac disease is the most serious form of gluten intolerance, but more and more people are becoming wheat-and/or gluten-intolerant.

In coeliac disease, the intestinal mucosal cells become sensitive to certain fractions of proteins in some grains, including wheat, rye, barley and oats, which means that these foods are poorly absorbed by the body. Gluten, a protein found in wheat, and its fraction (gliadin), are responsible for this sensitivity in coeliacs.

People who suffer from coeliac disease sometimes also suffer from lactose intolerance, and should therefore combine the gluten-free diet (see below) and the dairy-free diet (page 24).

THE GLUTEN-FREE DIET

Use the following as a guide to what you should eat and what you should avoid:

Meat, poultry and fish
Avoid these foods: All foods crumbed or dusted with wheat flour, or creamed; foods in which flour is used as the thickening agent; all foods with breadcrumbs added
Use instead: All fresh and frozen meat, poultry and fish

Milk and milk products
Avoid these foods: Drinks containing malt; ice cream or sorbet containing gluten stabilisers; Ovaltine, Milo and similar drinks
Use instead: All products except those listed above

Fruit and vegetables
Avoid these foods: All creamed or crumbed vegetables
Use instead: Fresh, frozen or canned fruit and vegetables, and fruit or vegetables juices

Starches and grains
Avoid these foods: Any products made from wheat, barley, rye or oats; commercially prepared bread mixes; scones, muffins and other wheat-flour baked products; bran flakes; macaroni, noodles and other pasta; malt
Use instead: Breads and cereals made from mealie meal, soya bean flour, rice flour, potato flour, puffed rice, cornflakes, potatoes or potato crisps, tortillas and tacos made from mealie meal (the American 'corn' is actually maize or mealies, and these products are made from yellow mealie meal)

Drinks and other foods
Avoid these foods: Beer, ale, rye whiskey, commercial salad dressings, distilled white vinegar, soy sauce, products containing hydrolised vegetable protein, prepared mustard, commercial sauces
Use instead: Wine, brandy, soft drinks, spices, herbs
Notes:
● Grains that may be included on gluten-free diets include corn (mealies) and rice.
● Substitutes for wheat flour are potato flour, mealie meal, rice flour, buckwheat, tapioca or soya bean flour.

GLOSSARY

Allergy: Hypersensitivity to a substance that causes the body to react to any contact with that substance. Hay fever, for example, is an allergic response to pollen.

Allergen: A substance, usually a protein, which can trigger an allergic response. All kinds of substances can be potential allergens, from pollen to perfume, dust mites to food.

Anaphylactic shock: A severe, often life-threatening, allergic reaction to a substance.

Antibodies: Large proteins produced in response to antigens, which then deactivate the antigens.

Antigen: A substance foreign to the body that will cause the formation of antibodies, or an inflammatory reaction, from immune system cells.

Food allergy: An allergic reaction to foods, involving an immune response, i.e. the body fights the 'intruder'; for example, swelling of throat tissue making breathing difficult, as a response to eating shellfish or eggs in a sensitive person. It is also called a food hypersensitive reaction.

Food intolerance: An adverse response to a food or food additive that does *not* involve the immune system; for example, gluten intolerance.

Gluten, a protein found in wheat, is responsible for sensitivity to wheat products. Gluten is important in yeast baking; when flour is kneaded with yeast it develops the gluten, which helps in the rising of the dough and gives the 'framework' to breads, rolls and loaves.

Alcohol, drugs and nutrition

Both alcohol and drugs interact with our nutritional status, and excessive use can pose serious threats to health.

ALCOHOL AND NUTRITION

In many cases, alcohol addiction leads to a poor nutritional status, which means that our bodies don't get the nutrients they need to function properly. Alcohol is high in energy, delivering 30 kilojoules per gram, and the more sugar there is in a drink, the higher the energy content will be. But these are 'empty' kilojoules, because they don't deliver any nutrients to our bodies; only energy from sugar and alcohol.

(Remember, if you're on a weight-loss diet, then you will have to include the kilojoules contained in any alcohol you consume in each day's total energy intake.)

Alcohol interferes with our bodies' ability to ingest, digest, absorb and metabolise nutrients and to excrete the excess, and is directly toxic to the liver.

The health risks associated with a high alcohol intake include:
- Cancer of the breast, colon, mouth, throat, oesophagus and lungs.
- Damage to the central nervous system, which is particularly sensitive to alcohol, resulting in 'the shakes'.
- Alcohol promotes *excessive* excretion of water by the kidneys; remember, however, that drinking a lot of water will help control the excretion of water by the kidneys.
- The most common damage is to the liver, which results in many side effects and can lead to diseases such as cirrhosis of the liver (page 48) and pancreatitis.
- Pregnant women who drink alcohol run the risk of bearing a child with Foetal Alcohol Syndrome, which results in multiple inborn defects.
- A high alcohol intake is also associated with hypertension, which can lead to heart disease (page 41).
- See also alcohol and the diabetic (page 54).

A sensible attitude to alcohol is to drink in moderation: no more than two drinks a day for men, and one for women (see standard portions for drinks, page 54). In fact, some research suggests that a *moderate* intake of alcohol may reduce the risk of cardiovascular disease because it raises the HDL cholesterol levels in the blood and helps prevent clot formation.

DRUGS AND NUTRITION
Regularly taking drugs, medicinally or otherwise, can have a serious impact on health, and can lead to serious drug/nutrient interactions, such as malabsorption of nutrients or decreased effectiveness of medication. Always follow the directions for use given on the packaging, or your doctor's instructions.

One cause for concern is that taking some drugs medicinally can lead to a patient becoming dependent on them, but if you follow your doctor's instructions this shouldn't happen.

Certain drugs, if abused, may have a severe impact on your nutritional status. The following are some examples:
- *Amphetamines* (see Glossary) decrease appetite and delay the onset of hunger, although a tolerance to the drug eventually develops.
- *Cocaine* leads to loss of appetite.
- *Codeine* leads to loss of appetite, if used regularly.
- *Marijuana* (dagga) is reported to enhance appetite in some people, while others lose weight and their appetites.
- With constant use, *methadone* leads to weight loss.

A wise course of action would be to check the side effects of prescribed and over-the-counter drugs with your doctor or pharmacist, and to supplement nutrients if you have to take medication on a regular basis. Check which nutrients you need to supplement with your doctor or pharmacist.

GLOSSARY

Amphetamines are used medicinally, mainly for their stimulant action on the central nervous system. They can have unpleasant or dangerous side effects and can lead to drug dependence.

Analgesic drugs are used to control pain.

Antibiotics: A group of medicines used to treat infections.

Weight management

Our bodies need energy to perform vital functions such as breathing and digesting food, as well as for our active lifestyles. Where does it get this energy?

To put it simply, to generate energy our bodies burn up (metabolise, see also page 8) the energy nutrients – carbohydrates, protein and fats – we take in through our food. What becomes of these nutrients in the body is extremely important, because it helps us understand why we lose, gain or maintain weight.

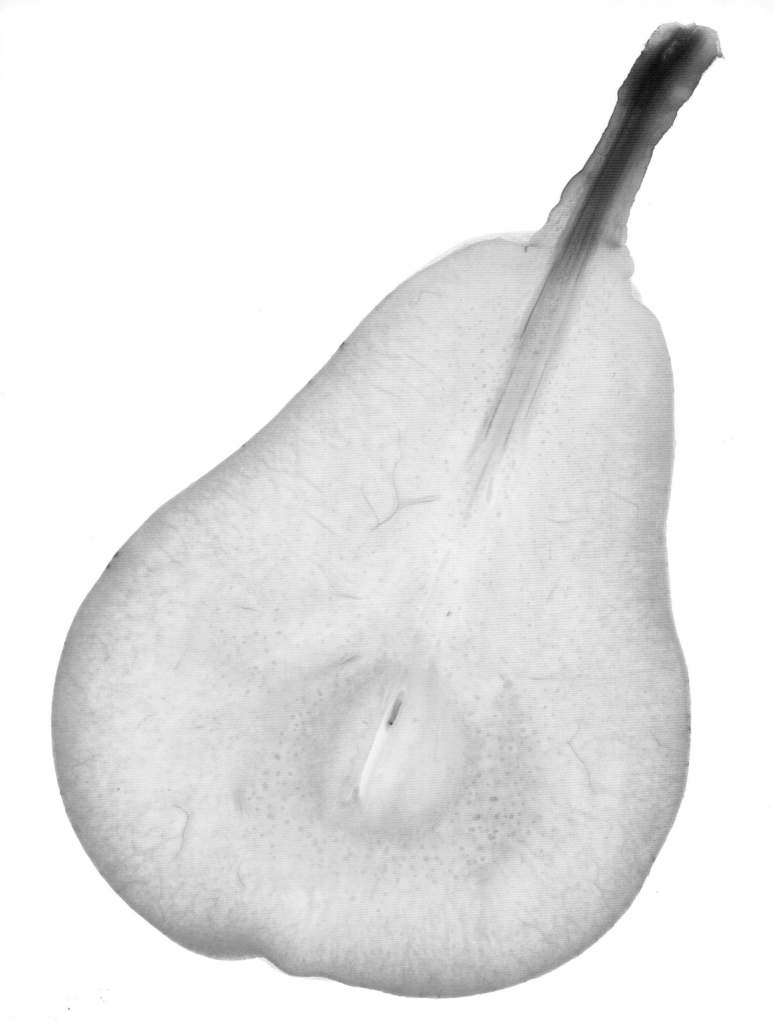

In the average body, the taking in and expending of energy usually balance each other, but some people eat too much and become fat; others eat too little and become thin.

When we take in more energy than we expend, much of the excess is stored as body fat. The bad news is that fat can be made from an excess of *any* energy-yielding nutrient that we eat. Excess energy from alcohol is also stored as body fat. Fat cells enlarge as they fill with fat, and our bodies' fat-storing capacity seems to be able to expand indefinitely.

Surplus *carbohydrates*, in the form of glucose, is first stored in the muscles and liver (as glycogen), but if these stores are full and the glucose is not used for energy, any excess is stored as fat. The same happens with any excess *proteins* and *fats* we take in. Fats, in particular, contribute very easily to our bodies' fat stores.

Our bodies expend energy all the time; even when we're asleep and totally relaxed, the cells of many organs are hard at work. This cellular work represents about two-thirds of the total energy we expend in a day. The other third is expended on the work our muscles do voluntarily during waking hours.

Fasting – such as when we're on a too-restricted weight-loss diet – means that we *voluntarily* stop eating food, whereas starvation means stopping eating involuntarily. The problem is that the body makes no distinction between the two; metabolically speaking, fasting and starvation are identical.

So when we fast, it means that we are living on our bodies' stored carbohydrates, fats and proteins. Our bodies are forced to draw on their reserves of carbohydrate and fat and, within a day or so, on the vital protein tissues as well. Low blood glucose concentrations are a signal to our bodies to break down more stored fat.

As fasting continues, our bodies reduce their energy output (**metabolic rate**, see Glossary) and conserve fat. Because our metabolism has slowed down, fat loss falls to a bare minimum. So, although weight loss during fasting may be quite dramatic, *fat* loss may actually be less than it is when some food, at least, is supplied.

Although our bodies adapt to fasting in order to maintain life over a long period, there are some hazards:
- Lean tissue (muscles) degenerates.
- Resistance to disease is reduced.
- Body temperature drops.
- The electrolyte (salt and water) balance is disturbed.

Fasting may be dangerous if we want to lose weight. Over a long period, a diet that's only moderately restricted in energy intake (through the energy-providing nutrients we eat) can actually promote a greater rate of weight loss, a faster rate of fat loss, and the retention of more lean tissue than a severely restricted fast.

HOW MUCH BODY FAT IS TOO MUCH?

What your ideal percentage of body fat is depends partly on you. A man, for example, may have 10 to 25 percent body fat, while a woman's may be 18 to 32 percent. For many athletes, a lower than average percentage of body fat may be ideal; just enough fat to provide energy, insulate and protect the body, assist in nerve impulse transmissions and support normal hormone activity, but not so much as to add excess weight for the muscles to carry. The most important criterion for 'appropriate' fatness is your health.

CAUSES OF OVERWEIGHT AND OBESITY

Simply put, excess body fat accumulates when we take in more food energy than we expend. It is likely, however, that obesity has many interrelated causes, of which the following are the most important:
- *Genetics*. If both your parents are obese, the chances that you will be overweight are high – some researchers put this as high as 80 percent. Genetics may influence the way your body stores energy, as well as how much energy your body expends.

  The differences in metabolic rate among individuals are more complex than can be explained by age, gender and body composition alone, and a low metabolic rate is a major risk factor for gaining weight.

  Researchers have also discovered a gene in humans called the 'obesity gene', which appears to act on the hypothalamus and influences appetite and energy balance. Exactly how this gene works is, however, still being investigated.
- *Emotional factors* may also play a role in overeating, as well as in the kinds of foods indulged in. Yearnings, cravings and addictions can express themselves in your eating behaviour; for example,

you may eat to compensate for boredom or rejection, or to ward off depression. (See Eating disorders, page 33.)

- *Physical inactivity.* Getting enough exercise is an important part of nutritional health. You have to be physically active if you are to eat enough food to obtain all the nutrients your body needs, without gaining weight. So it follows that if you are physically inactive, but still eat the foods you need to obtain all the necessary nutrients, you will gain weight.

Like all other 'causes' of obesity, inactivity on its own fails to explain the condition fully. Genetics, fat cell development, **set point** (see Glossary) and overeating all offer possible – but still incomplete – explanations. What is most likely is that obesity has different causes and combinations of causes in different people. Some of these can be controlled; some may be beyond anyone's control.

One view that has been gaining ground is that obesity is no one's 'fault', and is not caused by undisciplined gluttony.

Today, treating overweight and controlling weight focus more on obtaining optimal health than on creating an unrealistic weight loss goal.

HEALTH RISKS

Being overweight can increase the risk for hypertension (high blood pressure) and strokes, and cardiovascular disease and diabetes mellitus may be precipitated in genetically susceptible people who are also overweight. The risk for contracting some cancers – for example, breast cancer and colon cancer – may also increase in overweight people.

Some other problems overweight people may encounter include osteoarthritis, gout, gall bladder disease, respiratory problems, and complications during pregnancy or surgery.

It's thought that fat deposits in the central abdominal area of your body, rather than being fat all over, is likely to lead to diabetes, strokes, hypertension and coronary artery disease.

TREATING OVERWEIGHT AND OBESITY

The way you set about trying to lose weight could be risky; some weight-loss diets and treatments are healthy, but many more may be ineffective in the long run and could be dangerous.

Poor treatment choices include:

- Diet pills. Although some over-the-counter pills intended to suppress your appetite or increase your metabolic rate may have some temporary benefits, they shouldn't be taken for too long as they can affect your metabolic rate adversely and can be addictive. Your best course of action is to have a medical check-up and to combine medical treatment with a balanced eating plan.
- Diuretics used to eliminate 'excess' water from your body may be dangerous and can lead to dehydration (see page 21) and a mineral imbalance. Only water is lost; not fat.
- Fad diets are frequently based on false or exaggerated theories of weight loss, and are often lacking in energy and nutrients. They may offer some short-term weight loss success, but results will not be permanent, and some are more dangerous to your health than obesity itself. Your best course of action is to follow a balanced, kilojoule-restricted eating plan. Ask your doctor or nutritionist for advice.
- Laxatives, often sold as herbal weight-loss remedies, could cause nausea, vomiting, diarrhoea and the malabsorption of nutrients.
- Herbal products. Many alternative therapies (page 11) may be both effective and safe if used correctly. But remember that herbs are also drugs, and may interfere with, or maximise the effects of, other herbs or medication.
- Low-carbohydrate diets. If your body doesn't get sufficient carbohydrate, it cannot use its fat stores as it should. High blood cholesterol levels (because these diets are often very high in protein), mineral imbalances, low blood sugar levels and so on are other physiological problems that may accompany so-called 'low-carb' diets.
- Very low energy diets are designed to provide about 3 600 kJ, 1 gram of high-quality protein per kilogram of body weight, little or no fat, and a minimum of 50 g carbohydrate. This is not enough to ensure that there is enough protein to build muscles, or for other bodily processes.

Unfortunately, our bodies respond to severe energy restriction as if we were starving; they save energy and prepare to regain weight at the first opportunity, so the minute you go off your diet, you will start regaining weight (see Weight cycling). In addition, several changes occur as a result of living on such a low energy intake; for example, in hormone concentrations, fluid and electrolyte balances, metabolic rate and organ functions. Common side effects include headaches, fatigue, nausea, hair loss and dry skin. For these reasons, such diets should only be followed for a limited period (no more than four months), and *only* under medical supervision.

LONG-TERM STRATEGIES FOR WEIGHT LOSS

Successful weight loss is not determined by weight-for-height tables, but by the reduction of risk for diseases. Whether your goal is health or fitness, your expectations must be reasonable; unrealistic targets will just frustrate you and will probably result in failure.

No particular diet is magical; what you should be aiming for is a sensible eating plan you can follow for the rest of your life, which is what you will have to do if you want to keep off the weight you've lost.

Here are a couple of pointers:

- Be realistic in determining your energy intake. Most adults shouldn't eat less than 5 000 kJ a day in order to get all the nutrients they need from their food. To lose weight while conserving lean muscle – which should be your goal – calculate your daily energy intake at about 80 kJ per 1 kg of your current weight. So, for example, if you weigh 70 kg, your daily energy intake should total 5 600 kJ. Simply put, to lose 500 g a week, you need to cut 2 000 kJ a day.
- Using the Dietary guidelines for healthy people (page 10), choose foods you like and that are readily available. This will make it easier to follow your eating plan. See also Suggested eating patterns for different energy (kJ) intakes (page 32).
- Concentrate on complex carbohydrates such as grains, legumes, vegetables and fruit. Fat on food will add fat to your body, so cut off all visible fat from meat and use low-fat dairy products.
- Cut down on concentrated sweets and alcohol, and drink plenty of water.
- Eat small portions of food at each meal, and eat at the table. Remember to eat slowly, savouring the food and chewing it well.

- Your attitude to your weight-loss programme is extremely important. Think of it as an eating plan for life; if you think of it as a reducing diet, you're likely to be tempted to abandon it.
- For best results combine exercise with your weight-loss programme.

Exercising combined with a weight-loss programme has numerous benefits, including:

- An increase in energy expenditure, from the exercise itself and also from a rise in your metabolic rate
- Strengthened muscles and improved agility
- Appetite control, especially of the kind that arises from boredom and depression – if you're tempted to eat but you're not really hungry, exercise will help
- A reduction in stress, and control of eating in response to this
- Physical and psychological wellbeing
- Improved self-esteem.

WEIGHT CYCLING

Weight cycling, or 'yo-yo' dieting, is the endlessly repeated round of weight loss and regained weight. Usually, each bout of dieting is followed by a rebound of a higher weight than before. Such fluctuations in body weight appear to increase the risk of chronic diseases, so maintaining a stable weight (even if it's overweight) may be less harmful to your health.

WEIGHT-CONTROL TIPS

- Keep a daily record of what you eat and your exercise.
- Avoid buying 'problem' foods: those that are high in fat or sugar.
- Don't shop when you're hungry; you'll be tempted to buy foods you shouldn't eat.
- Make a shopping list and stick to it. Avoid impulse buying.
- Always sit down at a table to eat; snacking while you're standing in front of the refrigerator can quickly pile up the kilojoules.
- Stick to your plate of food, and clean plates as soon as you've finished. Store leftovers so that you're not tempted to nibble.
- Make small portions of food appear larger by serving them on smaller plates.

- Arrange food attractively on the plate to tempt your appetite and prevent a feeling of deprivation.
- Don't go without food for too long; eating regular meals is the way to go. If you're too hungry or too tired, you'll be tempted to nibble on high-fat or high-sugar snacks.
- Eat your meal slowly, pausing from time to time, to really savour your food.
- Don't read or watch television while you're eating; not only is sitting cramped over a plate bad for your digestion, but you'll be tempted to nibble too.
- Listen to your body and if it tells you it's full, don't force yourself to eat what's on your plate, just because it's there. Mums should also not finish off the food their children leave on their plates to avoid waste; it's amazing how many kilojoules those few mouthfuls can add!
- Physical activity doesn't only mean exercising. Moving around more instead of being a couch potato, flexing your muscles and stretching your back are all good for your physical condition.
- One way to ensure you keep to your healthy eating plan is to plan little rewards for yourself – *not* food! You might take a trip to the theatre, for instance, or buy yourself pretty underwear, when a milestone weight is reached.
- It often helps to go on a healthy weight-loss programme with a group of people, because you bolster one another's commitment when it's flagging. Join a weight-loss club in your area, or start one yourself.

FOOD GROUP	ENERGY LEVEL (kJ)						
	5 040	6 300	7 560	8 400	9 240	10 920	12 600
Bread, cereal, rice, pasta (portion: 1 slice bread, 125 ml [½ cup] cereal, rice)	6*	7*	8*	9*	11*	13*	15*
Meat & meat alternatives	120 g	150 g	180 g	180 g	180 g	210 g	240 g
Vegetables (portion: 125 ml [½ cup] cooked, 250 ml [1 cup] raw)	3*	4*	5*	5*	5*	6*	6*
Fruit (portion: 1 whole)	2*	3*	4*	4*	4*	5*	6*
Milk & milk products (portion [fat-free]: 250 ml [1 cup] milk or yoghurt, 30 g cottage cheese)	2*	2*	2*	3*	3*	3*	3*
Fats (portion: 5 ml [1 tsp] margarine or substitute)	3*	5*	6*	7*	8*	10*	12*

* = portions

SUGGESTED EATING PATTERNS FOR DIFFERENT ENERGY (kJ) INTAKES

The table on page 32 gives you some idea of the number of food portions (or the weight of a protein portion) you should select from each food group, to ensure a balanced eating plan for your targeted kilojoule intake. Remember, if you add extra sugar, butter or oil, the kilojoule count will rise.

The bottom line is: to ensure that you don't put on weight, you need to exercise, and in this way balance energy expended with the energy intake of nutrients your body needs for you to be healthy.

STRATEGIES FOR WEIGHT GAIN

Some people are naturally thin, and may want to gain a little weight. The same basic principles apply for weight gain as for weight loss: eat a healthy, balanced diet and also exercise.

People who need to gain weight are often picky eaters, and become so involved in what they're doing that they completely forget to eat.

If you want to gain weight, the temptation is to eat only high-energy foods but this is not a good strategy because, even though you will gain weight, it will only be fat. The ideal is to build lean tissue (muscle), not fat. The way to do this is to increase your energy intake by about 3 000 kJ to 4 200 kJ a day, above your normal energy needs, which will be enough to build muscle and have energy available for physical activity.

Here are some tips for gaining weight in a healthy way:
- Choose energy-dense foods such as full-fat milk and dairy products, medium-fat meats, fruit juice, avocadoes, olives and nuts. Eating too much saturated fat is never healthy, however, so choose olive oil and other plant oils for cooking and dressings.
- Make sure you eat at least three meals a day, and have healthy snacks in between and before you go to bed.
- Try to eat larger portions of food, and – as for those who want to lose weight – eat at the table, not in front of the TV.
- If you still find that you aren't gaining weight as you wish, try taking a weight-gain supplement, available from pharmacies, in a glass of milk or in soup.

GLOSSARY

Metabolic rate: The rate at which our bodies burn up the nutrients we take in, to generate energy.

Set point: The point at which your weight will stabilise.

Eating disorders

Eating disorders are generally described as a disturbance in eating behaviour that jeopardises physical and psychological health.

Although there are numerous unspecified eating behaviours, such as restricted eating, bingeing and purging, two distinct eating disorders are cause for concern. These are anorexia nervosa and bulimia nervosa.

Girls and young women, in particular, are likely to suffer from these two disorders. Anorexia and bulimia sometimes overlap, they can appear in the same person, and one can lead to the other.

ANOREXIA NERVOSA

This eating disorder is characterised by a fear of becoming fat and the refusal of food. People who suffer from anorexia have such an excessive preoccupation with weight loss that it becomes an extreme danger to their health and even their lives.

Excessive pressure to be thin is at least partly to blame. Some adolescent girls (and sometimes adolescent boys) make being thin their ideal and become dissatisfied with their body weight, perceiving a healthy body and a normal weight as being 'too fat'.

So they try severe, unhealthy and often dangerous diets to lose their 'excess' weight which often leads to a cycle of **bingeing** (see Glossary) and purging from which they find it difficult to escape. It becomes more and more difficult to lose weight because of this (see Weight cycling, page 31), psychological problems often get worse and the likelihood of developing an eating disorder becomes greater.

Athletes and dancers are often at risk, because they have to meet stringent weight and shape requirements. When young athletes and dancers reach adolescence, their bodies frequently change shape and they become desperate to 'undo' these changes. As a result, they are especially prone to developing psychological problems triggered by their weight and shape. They may try extreme methods to lose weight, such as excessive dieting, diet pills, fasting, vomiting, or using saunas and steam baths.

Physical problems, such as amenorrhoea (absence of at least three consecutive menstruation periods) and osteoporosis (page 19) may also occur, which in turn lead to low blood estrogen levels, infertility and bone mineral losses – which could lead to bone fractures.

Good nutrition is an important facet of the training of athletes and dancers, and they should remember that eating disorders impair physical performance.

DIAGNOSING ANOREXIA NERVOSA

There are two types of anorexics: those who follow a self-induced fast, and refuse to eat even minimal quantities of food; and those who regularly binge and purge afterwards.

These are the criteria for diagnosing anorexia:
- A refusal to maintain their body weight at, or above, the minimum normal weight for their age and height; in other words, a body weight of less than 85 percent of what would be expected for their age and height.
- An intense fear of gaining weight, or becoming fat, even if underweight.
- Body weight or shape seen as being excessive and unacceptable, *on their own evaluation*; and denial of the seriousness of the current low body weight.
- Disturbance in the menstrual cycle of girls past puberty, because of the extreme loss of body tissue. If there is no menstruation for three consecutive months, it is a cause for concern.

COMBATING ANOREXIA

Here are some tips:
- Establish a *realistic* goal weight, based on body shape and build.
- Set *realistic* targets for losing weight or fat tissue. Focus on health instead, and exercise regularly (but not excessively!).
- Never restrict food portions to below the quantities suggested in the Dietary guidelines for healthy people (page 10).
- Eat meals regularly, so that you won't get so hungry or desperate for food that you're tempted to binge.

- Start a weight-maintenance support group; it's always easier in the company of others with the same goal.

TREATING ANOREXIA NERVOSA

Treatment is tricky, because the anorexic often denies that she has a problem, and therefore thinks she does not need treatment.

The best course of action is to take a multidisciplinary approach, with doctors, psychologists, dieticians and family therapists forming part of the team during the treatment. What is most important is that the patient must have confidence in all the people working with her.

The treatment has to be individualised and counselling often has to continue for a long time. High-risk patients may have to be hospitalised, and some may need to be force-fed to save their lives which, in turn, can lead to severe psychological trauma.

Unfortunately, there is a high relapse rate, especially once the anorexic has to confront the stresses of life again.

BULIMIA NERVOSA

Typically, sufferers from bulimia nervosa, a condition characterised by compulsive overeating, will alternate episodes of bingeing with severe self-starvation or self-induced vomiting, and take laxatives or diuretics to – in their minds – 'undo the damage'.

Unlike anorexics, bulimics are aware of the consequences of their behaviour; they know it is abnormal and are deeply ashamed of it. They feel inadequate and unable to control their eating, which leads to depression.

If the depression deepens, bulimics may seek solace in drugs, alcohol or other depressive behaviours. It is estimated, for example, that as many as 50 percent of women who are bulimics are also alcohol-dependent.

A typical binge takes place in secret, often at night, and lasts for an hour or more. The food indulged in typically contains little fibre or water, has a smooth texture and is high in sugar and fat so that it is easy to consume vast quantities rapidly, with little chewing.

Bingeing and purging have serious health and physical consequences: fluid and electrolyte imbalances; irritation and infection of the pharynx, oesophagus and salivary glands as a result of the vomiting; tooth erosion and dental caries (tooth decay). In extreme cases,

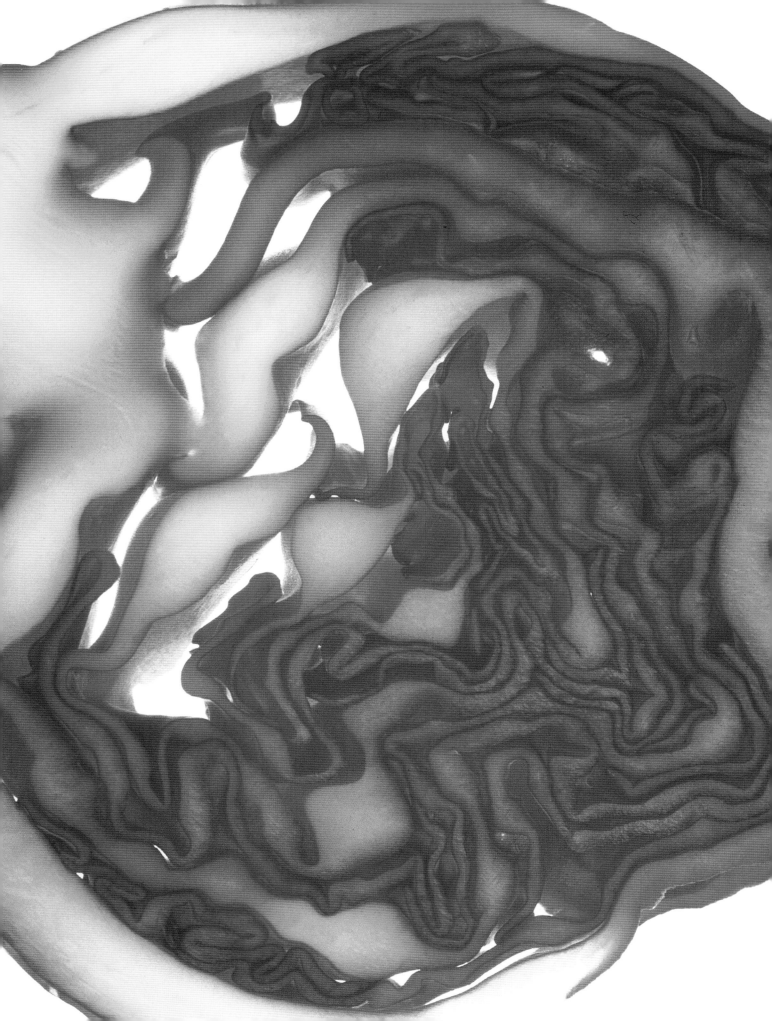

the oesophagus may rupture or tear, and if potassium stores are depleted, heart failure can result.

DIAGNOSING BULIMIA NERVOSA

There are two types of bulimics: those who regularly engage in self-induced vomiting or the misuse of laxatives, diuretics or enemas; and those who don't regularly use such purging methods but display other inappropriate behaviours, such as fasting or excessive exercise.

The criteria for diagnosing bulimia nervosa include:
- Recurrent episodes of **bingeing** (see Glossary)
- Resorting to self-induced vomiting, enemas, laxatives and diuretics, or excessive exercise, in order to prevent weight gain
- Binge-eating and purging episodes occurring on average at least twice a month, for a period of at least three months
- Self-evaluation unduly influenced by body shape and weight.

COMBATING BULIMIA NERVOSA

Here are some tips:
- Plan meals and snacks and keep a food diary, detailing what you eat, how much, and when.
- Avoid finger foods; always use cutlery when you eat.
- Choose warm foods, which will lead to a feeling of fullness and satisfaction.
- Choose whole-grain and high-fibre breads and cereals as well as vegetables and fruit to prolong eating time and maximise food bulk.
- Always sit down to eat meals, and don't read or watch TV while eating.
- Buy smaller containers of tempting foods such as ice cream and yoghurt.

TREATING BULIMIA NERVOSA

As in the case of anorexia nervosa, a team approach provides the most effective treatment. The main goal is to help the bulimic gain control over her eating habits, and learn to eat nutritious foods in order to combat hunger.

GLOSSARY

Bingeing: Eating, over a relatively short period, a quantity of food that is definitely larger than most people would eat during a similar period, and under similar circumstances. There is also a sense of lack of control over eating during the episode; a feeling that you cannot stop eating or control what, or how much, you are eating.

The digestive tract

Many ailments and diseases affect the digestive tract, and some are more serious than others.

HEARTBURN

A burning pain felt behind the breastbone is an indication of heartburn, a condition in which stomach acids irritate the oesophagus. Although not serious, it can be very unpleasant to suffer an attack of heartburn.

Some foods increase acid secretion in the stomach: fats, alcohol, caffeine (decaffeinated coffee, too!), chocolate, peppermint and spearmint are all likely culprits. Other foods might irritate the oesophagus – tomatoes and tomato sauce, for instance, as well as pepper and other spices, very hot or cold foods, and citrus fruits and juices. So the first step is to find out which food or drink causes the heartburn; keeping a diary of what you eat and your daily activities will help you isolate the cause.

Taking an over-the-counter antacid will neutralise the acidity in your stomach, as will antacids prescribed by your doctor to curb acid production and/or strengthen cardiac sphincter pressure. These medications must be taken with caution, as taking too many antacids could upset the mineral balance in your bones.

Here are some tips for combating heartburn:
- Eat small meals, and drink liquids an hour before or after meals to avoid distending your stomach.
- Have a relaxing meal, seated at the table, and make sure you eat slowly and chew food well to avoid swallowing air, which could distend your stomach.
- Avoid foods that might irritate the oesophagus.
- Being overweight tends to increase pressure in the

stomach, and often losing a little weight diminishes the discomfort.

- Don't wear tight-fitting clothes, which will add to the discomfort of heartburn.
- For the same reason, don't lie down for a nap immediately after eating a meal, and try not to bend over suddenly or too strenuously.
- Try raising the head of your bed or adding a pillow or two, to avoid putting pressure on your stomach while you sleep.
- Avoid, or cut down on, cigarettes; smoking can also add to the discomfort because of the air that is inhaled.

GASTRITIS

This very common ailment is characterised by the stomach lining becoming inflamed and painful. Symptoms include loss of appetite, nausea, vomiting and pain. Gastritis has a number of causes, and can be the result of taking too many tablets containing aspirin or other medications over a long period, alcohol abuse, food allergies, food poisoning, radiation therapy and infections.

To ease gastritis, doctors often prescribe a bland diet (page 38) that omits spices and other foods that might irritate the bowel further.

ULCERS

The open sores or lesions called ulcers may have many sites in the body, such as in the duodenum, but the most common one is a **peptic ulcer** (see Glossary), sited in the stomach.

Three major causes of ulcers have been identified: bacterial infection, the use of certain medication (especially anti-inflammatories), and excessive secretion of stomach acids.

Treatment of ulcers aims to relieve the pain, heal the ulcer and prevent a recurrence. Drugs are usually prescribed to treat the causes. Ulcers can be treated through diet: during the acute phase, a bland diet (page 38) is best, but after that the ulcer sufferer should follow a well-balanced eating plan, eat regularly and avoid any food or drink known to cause an irritation to the bowel.

IRRITABLE BOWEL SYNDROME (IBS)

This condition, often called a spastic colon, is not a disease but a syndrome and is characterised by abdominal pain, bloating and abnormal bowel movements. Diarrhoea, alternating with constipation, also occurs.

IBS is usually not life-threatening, even if it is painful. Making sure you obtain enough nutrients through what you eat, concentrating on high-fibre foods (see highfibre diet, page 38) and an ample intake of water (to balance the fibre) will help. Do *not*, however, follow a high-fat diet, and avoid caffeine, all sugars and alcohol.

The syndrome is linked to high stress levels, so relaxation and stress-reduction therapy often work wonders.

DIVERTICULITIS

Some people are prone to this condition, which affects the sac-like pouches in the walls of the colon. Symptoms range from mild bleeding to inflammation, excessive bleeding and, finally, obstruction of the colon.

Following a high-fibre diet (page 38) will benefit you if you're prone to diverticulitis, but note that if your diet has been low in fibre for many years, you should gradually ease into a high-fibre diet. If you have an acute flare-up of diverticulitis, you may need to follow a low-residue diet (page 38) until the symptoms clear up.

SPECIAL DIETS FOR DIGESTIVE TRACT PROBLEMS

A number of special diets may be prescribed for gastric ailments. These include liquid diets, soft diets, bland diets, low-residue diets, low-fibre diets and high-fibre diets.

LIQUID DIETS

These may be either a clear liquid diet or a full liquid diet, and may be prescribed for gastric ailments such as diarrhoea or following complete bowel rest, as well as after surgery of all kinds. Your doctor or dietician will give you a suitable diet plan to follow.

SOFT DIETS

A soft diet may be prescribed for indigestion, nausea, gastritis and diarrhoea. Soft diets provide soft but solid foods which are lightly seasoned and moderate or low in fibre, and which are easy to chew, digest and absorb. High-fibre foods, nuts, seeds, spicy foods, as well as foods which might produce gas – such as cabbage, broccoli, dried beans or peas, onions and garlic – must be omitted. (See also Foods that cause flatulence, page 39.) Meals are smaller, and more frequent.

These foods may be included in a soft diet: Tender and moist meats; fish or poultry; mild cheeses; creamy peanut butter; eggs; milk and milk products; cooked, or soft fresh fruit such as melons; fruit juices; soft-cooked vegetables (except those likely to cause flatulence); re- fined white or light rye bread; rolls or crackers; cooked or ready-to-eat cereals without nuts or seeds; mild condi- ments; salt; sugar; mildly seasoned broths or soups; non-alcoholic drinks; desserts without nuts, seeds or coconut.

BLAND DIETS

A bland diet excludes foods that will stimulate gastric acid secretion, irritate the stomach lining or cause indi- gestion. It may be prescribed for ulcers, nausea, heart- burn, hiatus hernia, gastritis and peptic ulcers.

Bland diets include all foods, except:
- Those that irritate the digestive tract
- Alcohol
- Caffeine and caffeine-containing drinks such as cola, some sports drinks and cocoa
- Decaffeinated coffee and tea
- Pepper, chilli and other spicy foods (which will cause discomfort but will not damage the stomach lining).

LOW-RESIDUE DIETS

The low-residue diet, like the low-fibre diet, is usually prescribed to restrict total stool volume, because it is least likely to obstruct a digestive tract narrowed by scarring, or in which movement is slow. The low- residue diet restricts all high-fibre foods, including veg- etables and fruit juices. Milk and milk products are also restricted. These diets are usually temporary, but if they're prescribed for longer periods, they must be sup- plemented with vitamins and minerals.

LOW-FIBRE DIETS

Like the low-residue diet, a low-fibre diet may be pre- scribed in an effort to restrict total stool volume. It allows tender meat, poultry, seafood and eggs, as well as refined breads, cereal, rice and pasta, but limits the types and serving portions of fruit and vegetables. Fruits allowed include cooked or canned peeled apples, apricots, peaches, bananas, cherries, naartjies, fruit juice, avocados and nuts; permitted vegetables are cooked squash, tomato purée and puréed cooked celery.

HIGH-FIBRE DIETS

High-fibre diets may be prescribed for irritable bowel syndrome (IBS) as well as for other gastric problems. If you're not used to eating a lot of fibre, introduce it grad- ually, and add high-fibre foods as your tolerance improves. You must also take sufficient fluid, because fibre attracts water as it moves through the intestine.

Foods for a high-fibre diet include: whole-grain breads and cereals; brown and wild rice; apples; berries; figs; paw- paw; prunes; pears; guavas; artichokes; broccoli; Brussels sprouts; raw carrots; legumes; sweet potatoes; turnips; peanut butter; popcorn.

Good ways of adding fibre to your diet include mix- ing high-fibre foods with other foods – for example, sprinkling bran flakes, wheat germ or raisins over cere- als, salads or vegetables and adding legumes (cooked dried peas and beans) to soups and mince dishes.

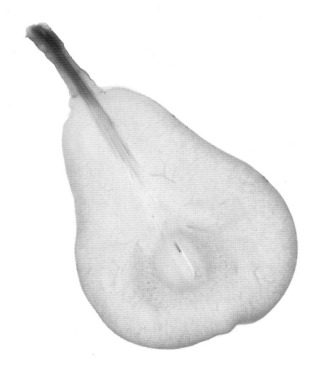

FOODS THAT CAUSE FLATULENCE

UNDIGESTED AND UNABSORBED DIETARY FIBRE, AS WELL AS
FOODS, MAY BE METABOLISED IN THE COLON AND PRODUCE
GAS IN THE PROCESS. UNABSORBED LACTOSE (MILK SUGAR)
MAY CAUSE GAS IN PEOPLE WHO ARE LACTOSE-INTOLERANT.
TO PREVENT FLATULENCE, CHEW YOUR FOOD PROPERLY, AND
DON'T TALK WHILE YOU EAT AS YOU MAY ALSO SWALLOW AIR –
WHICH CAN LEAD TO GAS FORMING. AVOID THESE FOODS AS
WELL:

- APPLES
- ASPARAGUS
- BEER
- BRAN
- BROCCOLI
- BRUSSELS SPROUTS
- CABBAGE
- CARBONATED DRINKS
- CAULIFLOWER
- CREAM SAUCES
- CUCUMBER
- FRIED FOODS
- FRUCTOSE
- GARLIC
- GRAVY
- HIGH-FAT MEATS
- HONEY
- LEGUMES (DRIED PEAS AND BEANS)
- MILK AND MILK PRODUCTS
- NUTS
- ONIONS
- PRUNES
- RADISHES
- RAISINS
- SORBITOL
- SOYA BEANS
- WHEAT

NUTRITION AND A COLOSTOMY

After surgery to remove a portion of the colon (large intestine), and the creating of a **stoma** (see Glossary), the patient will at first be put on a bland diet (page 38) to prevent obstructing the opening and to promote healing.

Other foods should be added to the diet as soon as possible, one at a time and in small quantities, to make sure that there are no problems.

Bear the following in mind if you have a stoma:

- Obstructions in the bowel can cause a lot of problems and severe pain. Prevent them by eliminating stringy foods or foods with tough skins such as uncooked dried fruit, nuts, and tough raw fruits. Chewing food well will also reduce the chances of an obstruction.
- Extra fluids are needed because less fluid is absorbed from the large intestine. There's no need to worry that fluids will cause diarrhoea; they don't, and the excess is excreted by the kidneys.
- **Diarrhoea** (see Glossary) may be a problem. Foods that will thicken the stool are apple sauce, bananas, cheese and starchy foods such as breads, rice and potatoes. Foods that may cause diarrhoea are raw apples, grapes and prunes, highly seasoned foods and caffeine. You'll learn by experience which foods you can and cannot eat.
- Gas and odours may be a problem. Avoid the gas-producing foods mentioned alongside, but once again, you will learn by your own experience which foods will cause gas. Foods that are thought to reduce odours include yoghurt, buttermilk and parsley.

GLOSSARY

Diarrhoea: Thin, runny stools.

Peptic ulcer: An erosion of the top layer of cells from the stomach lining, causing a burning sensation. Peptic ulcers are irritated by stomach acids, and the treatment is a bland diet that will not irritate the raw stomach lining.

Stoma: A surgically formed opening through which waste will be excreted, in patients who have had part of, or the entire, colon removed.

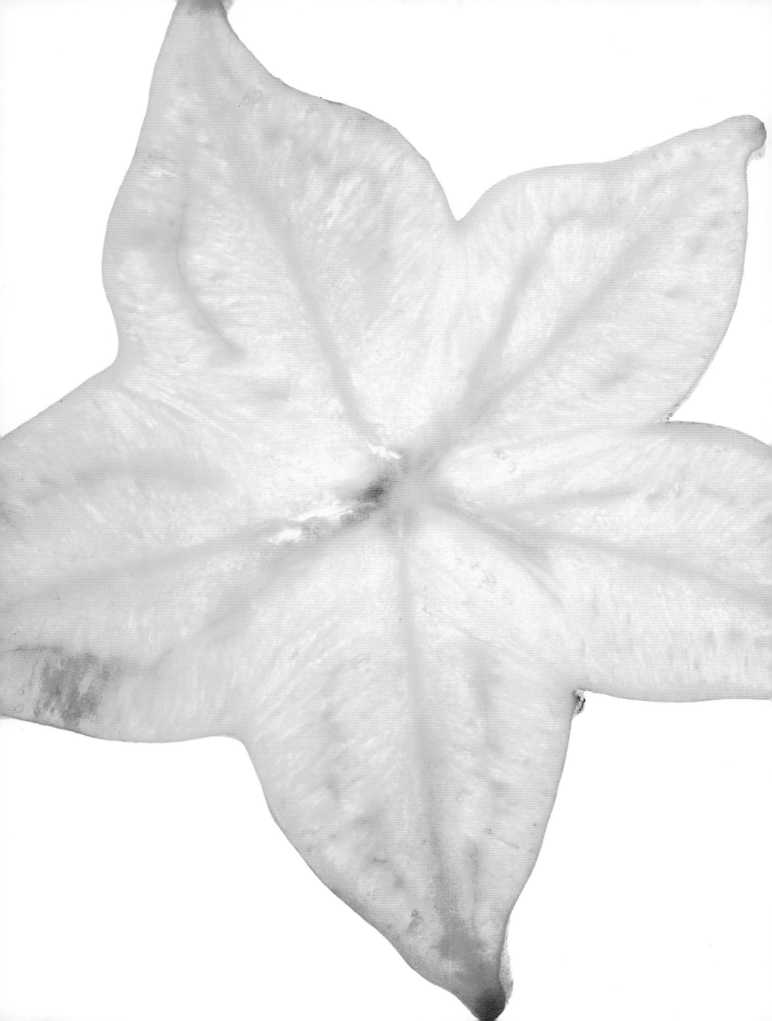

The heart and coronary diseases

Cardiovascular disease or CVD – a general term for all diseases of the heart and blood vessels – is one of the leading causes of death in the world today. The mortality rate in men aged 35 to 50 is three times higher than that for women of the same ages, but the incidence levels out after the age of 65.

The most common CVDs are heart diseases, such as **arteriosclerosis** (see Glossary) and **hypertension** (see Glossary), and **strokes** (see Glossary). Each has its own set of risk factors, and each condition aggravates the others.

The degenerative disease **atherosclerosis** (see Glossary) usually begins with the accumulation of soft fatty streaks, called plaque, along the inner lining of arterial walls, especially at branch points. The plaque may gradually enlarge and become hardened with calcium and connective tissue. As the plaque deposits become larger, they tend to obstruct the arteries, which leads to an increase in blood pressure.

Atherosclerosis also damages healthy tissues. When blood flow in the arteries feeding the heart is obstructed, coronary artery disease occurs. The heart muscle is damaged, resulting in pain and pressure in and around the area of the heart, a condition called **angina** (see Glossary). If the obstruction becomes extremely severe or if a blood clot lodges in a damaged artery and the blood flow to the heart is cut off, that area of the heart muscle dies, and a **heart attack** (see Glossary) results. When the blood flow to the brain is obstructed, a stroke may occur.

Blood clots form and dissolve in the blood all the time, but in atherosclerosis, clots form faster than they dissolve. A smaller clot may become lodged on plaque and gradually grow large enough to totally obstruct a blood vessel. This is called **thrombosis** (see Glossary). The gradual or sudden loss of blood flow to the portion of tissue affected robs the tissue of nutrients and oxygen, and the tissue may eventually die.

The heart has to create enough pressure to pump blood throughout the entire body. When the arteries are narrowed by disease, clots or plaque, or all of them, the blood flow is restricted and the heart has to work harder and generate more pressure to deliver the oxygen-rich blood to body tissues. The artery walls are damaged further by the increased blood pressure. Although atherosclerosis can invade any blood vessel, the coronary (heart) arteries are most often affected.

Preventive efforts focus on delaying or reversing the progression of existing plaque. Free radicals, which form in the body during the course of normal metabolism (page 8), may also play a part in the progression of plaque. Atherosclerosis treatment – to prevent or to treat the disease – aims to normalise blood fat levels and to minimise risk factors such as obesity, overweight and lack of physical activity.

RISK FACTORS FOR CORONARY DISEASE

The main risk factors for coronary disease are:

- Heredity. If there is a family history of heart attacks or sudden death before the age of 55 in a father or brother, or before 65 in the case of a mother or sister, it could be a strong indication of a hereditary factor – a warning to be really aware of the risk factors and to try to minimise them as much as possible
- High blood cholesterol levels
- Being male and over 45
- Being female and over the age of 55, and not on hormone replacement therapy
- High blood pressure
- Smoking
- Diabetes mellitus
- Too little exercise
- Stress
- Diet and eating habits that include a high fat intake.

Many of the risk factors are interrelated. Because what we eat influences body weight as well as the fat content of our blood, diet is one of the major modifiable factors. This is why amending our daily diet (eating plan) to eating foods lower in fats can help protect against coronary heart disease or CHD.

THE FATS IN FOOD

Dietary fats, meat and nuts contain variable amounts of fat, but two food groups – the milk, cheese and yoghurt group and the breads – may also contain fats. (See Dietary guidelines for healthy people, page 10.) The fat in full-cream milk, for example, is about 63 percent **saturated fats** (see Glossary), so choosing fat-free milk, yoghurt or cottage cheese will considerably reduce our intake of saturated and total fats.

In addition, fats may be added to food during processing or preparation. Added oil, butter, margarine, mayonnaise or cream can push up the fat content considerably.

Then there are the so-called 'hidden fats' in convenience foods, canned meats and other processed foods, fried foods and foods served with sauces.

Make no mistake: fats *do* have important functions in food preparation. They contribute flavour and aroma; they alter or influence the texture by adding creaminess, smoothness, moisture or crispness; they help make foods tender; and they carry fat-soluble vitamins, such as vitamin E. But if we eat too many fats, it can lead to increased **cholesterol** (see Glossary) and other fat levels in the blood, which in turn can cause plaque to build up in artery walls.

CHOLESTEROL AND BLOOD FATS

High blood cholesterol levels are often blamed as a high-risk factor for coronary heart disease.

The blood cholesterol linked to CHD risk is low-density lipoprotein cholesterol (LDL), which contributes to the formation of plaque on the artery walls. High-density lipoprotein (HDL) is believed to reduce the risk of heart disease. High **triglyceride** (see Glossary) levels are also linked to CHD.

All these factors may be altered considerably by following the correct eating plan, exercising regularly and more often, and making lifestyle changes.

PHYSICAL ACTIVITY

Being active can help speed up weight loss and loss of body fat. It will also strengthen the cardiovascular system, reduce high blood pressure and raise HDL cholesterol levels in the blood. In addition, exercise will improve glucose tolerance in people who have diabetes mellitus (page 50).

Exercise should be regular and it doesn't have to be too strenuous; even brisk walking for 30 minutes every day, or every second day, will make a big difference, and it will also improve mental health. Aerobic, endurance-type exercise is also recommended because it increases heart/lung capacity and will help control weight.

DIET THERAPY

Reducing LDL cholesterol levels in the blood is the main aim of diet therapy to prevent and treat coronary heart disease. This means controlling or reducing body weight (if overweight), and reducing the intake of total fats, saturated fats and dietary cholesterol (from foods).

Obesity is associated with high blood fat levels, hypertension and diabetes. Losing weight minimises the risk factors for heart disease and reduces high blood pressure, as well as LDL cholesterol and triglyceride levels.

The total amount of fats we eat every day should be no more than 30 percent of energy intake, and saturated fatty acids should be no more than a third of this percentage. For example, if our daily kJ (energy) intake is 10 000 kJ, fats should be no more than 80 g.

We should also include complex carbohydrates (fibre-rich foods) in our daily eating plan. They have cholesterol-lowering properties and, when used in a diet low in both total fats and saturated fats, the fibre found in foods such as oats, barley, fruits and vegetables may help to reduce blood fat levels even further.

A moderate consumption of alcohol (no more than two drinks a day, may also reduce the risk of CHD by raising HDL cholesterol levels and preventing clot formation.

Research has shown that people in Mediterranean countries have a lower incidence of cardiovascular disease. Mediterranean diets in general are low in saturated fats and high in **monounsaturated fats** (see Glossary), such as olive oil, as well as in dietary fibre, B-complex vitamins and antioxidants, such as beta-carotene, and vitamins C and E (page 9). The lifestyle in Mediterranean countries, however, is also different, which could have an effect on cardiovascular health.

CUT DOWN ON FATS

Fats can sneak into our daily diet through every food group. Here are some ways to control them:
Meat, fish and poultry
- Choose fish, poultry or lean pork or beef.
- Trim the visible fat from pork and beef, and remove skin from poultry before cooking
- Grill, pan-grill, roast, bake, stir-fry, stew or braise meat; don't fry. Where possible, place meat on a rack so that the fat can drain off during cooking.

- Use lean minced turkey or ostrich in recipes instead of beef mince.
- Brown minced meats without added fat, then drain off any fat excess.
- Refrigerate meat pan drippings and when it solidifies, remove the fat from the surface and use the remaining pan juices in recipes.
- Select canned tuna packed in water, or rinse oil-packed tuna in hot water to remove excess oil (fat).
- Thread plenty of vegetables and a few meat cubes on to kebab skewers and then grill.
- Create main dishes and casseroles by combining a little meat, fish or poultry with plenty of pasta, rice or vegetables.
- Make meatless pasta sauces and casseroles.
- Eat a meatless meal or two every day, but take care when using the milk and other food groups – some of them contain large amounts of fat.

Milk and cheese
- Drink fat-free, low-fat and reduced-fat milk instead of full-cream (whole) milk.
- Use fat-free, low-fat and reduced-fat cheeses, such as part-skim ricotta and low-fat mozzarella, instead of fat-rich cheeses such as Cheddar and blue-veined cheese.
- Enjoy fat-free frozen yoghurt or sorbet instead of ice cream for dessert.

Fruit and vegetables
- Imported butter-flavoured granules, available at certain supermarkets, may be used on cooked vegetables instead of butter or margarine.
- Use fat-free yoghurt or salad dressing instead of sour cream, mayonnaise, cheese or other sauces over vegetables and in casseroles.
- Select fat-free or low-fat (low-oil) mayonnaise or salad dressings, or use herbs, lemon juice and spices instead.
- Add a little water to thick, commercial salad dressings to dilute the amount of oil (fat) in each serving.
- Eat at least two vegetables (in addition to a salad) with your main meal.
- Snack on raw vegetables or fruit instead of high-fat foods such as potato crisps and biscuits.
- Enjoy fresh fruit for dessert.

Bread and cereals
- Use sucrose-free fruit spreads or jam on bread instead of butter or margarine.
- Select breads, rolls, cereals or crackers low in fat; for example, bagels instead of croissants.

LOW-FAT COOKING

- USE NONSTICK PANS OR SAUCEPANS, OR BRUSH THEM LIGHTLY WITH COOKING OIL.
- PREPARE SOUP OR STEWS THE DAY BEFORE, ALLOW THEM TO COOL COMPLETELY AND SPOON OFF THE FAT THAT SETTLES ON THE SURFACE BEFORE REHEATING AND SERVING.
- COOK VEGETABLES UNTIL JUST TENDER, BY STEAMING THEM IN VERY LITTLE WATER OR IN A STEAMER OVER BOILING WATER.
- USE 2 EGG WHITES INSTEAD OF EACH WHOLE EGG CALLED FOR IN RECIPES.
- USE HALF THE MARGARINE, BUTTER OR OIL CALLED FOR IN A RECIPE (THE MINIMUM AMOUNT OF FAT FOR MUFFINS AND QUICK BREADS IS 15-30 ML [1-2 TBSP] PER 250 ML [1 CUP] OF FLOUR; FOR CAKES AND COOKIES IT'S 30 ML [2 TBSP] PER 250 ML [1 CUP] OF FLOUR).
- SELECT WHIPPED OR LITE TYPES OF MARGARINE OR CREAM CHEESE, OR BUTTER/MARGARINE MIXES SUCH AS BUTRO, TO SERVE WITH MEALS; THEY CONTAIN HALF THE FAT AND KILOJOULES OF THE STANDARD TYPES OF MARGARINE AND BUTTER.
- USE WINE, LEMON JUICE OR DEFATTED PAN JUICES INSTEAD OF BUTTER OR MARGARINE WHEN COOKING.
- STIR-FRY IN VERY LITTLE OIL; ADD MOISTURE AND FLAVOUR WITH FAT-FREE PAN JUICES, TOMATO JUICE OR WINE INSTEAD.
- VARY COLOURS, TEXTURES AND TEMPERATURES OF FOODS AND COMPLEMENT THE MEAL WITH GARNISHES.
- USE LOW-FAT YOGHURT INSTEAD OF MAYONNAISE OR SOUR CREAM, OR COMBINE LOW-FAT YOGHURT WITH MAYONNAISE TO REDUCE ITS OIL (FAT) CONTENT.

CLEVER CHOICES

- FRESH VEGETABLES AND SALADS
- FRESH FRUIT, WITHOUT ADDED SUGAR
- OLIVE OIL, IN MODERATE QUANTITIES
- WHOLE-WHEAT BREAD AND RUSKS
- LOW-FAT OR FAT-FREE MILK AND CHEESE
- A GLASS OF RED WINE INSTEAD OF OTHER ALCOHOLIC DRINKS.

- CHOOSE TWO STARTERS RATHER THAN A LARGE MAIN DISH.
- ORDER GRILLED MEAT OR FISH.
- CHOOSE DISHES CONTAINING LOW-FAT PULSES, SUCH AS BEANS AND LENTILS; A SMALLER QUANTITY MAKES YOU FEEL FULL AND THEY ALSO ADD A DELICIOUS FLAVOUR.
- ORDER SAUCES SEPARATELY AND USE THE MINIMUM QUANTITY.
- ORDER A BAKED POTATO RATHER THAN CHIPS OR ROAST POTATOES – AND EAT IT WITH LOW-FAT YOGHURT (OR WITHOUT ANY TOPPING AT ALL) INSTEAD OF BUTTER OR SOUR CREAM.
- APPROACH THE CHEESE BOARD WITH CAUTION; PLENTY OF FATS LURK THERE!

SODIUM AND HEALTH

Salt, or sodium chloride, is a mineral made up of approximately 40 percent sodium and 60 percent chloride. It occurs naturally in foods, mainly meat, fish and dairy products.

Sodium is essential for good health; it is the principal **electrolyte** (see Glossary) in the body's extracellular fluid (fluid around the cells) and the primary regulator of extracellular fluid volume. We get thirsty when the blood concentration of sodium rises, and have to drink water or other fluids to make sure that our bodies' sodium-to-water ratio is restored to normal. Sodium is also essential to allow muscle contraction and neural (nerve) transmission to take place.

The ability of sodium (or rather the salt that contains it) to draw liquid from any matter or foodstuff to which it is added is well-known, and the same thing happens in our bodies. When our bodies contain too much sodium, it is not eliminated; body cells simply collect more fluid, which eventually places an extra burden on the heart and kidneys.

Sodium contributes to hypertension or high blood pressure in susceptible people and it is thought that susceptibility may increase with deficiencies in potassium, calcium and magnesium. High blood pressure is closely related to our chances of contracting coronary heart disease. In addition, scientific evidence points to high blood pressure being the strongest risk factor for a stroke.

There is also a good deal of evidence to suggest that a high sodium intake causes the body to excrete calcium from the bones, which reduces bone density and can lead to **osteoporosis** (see Glossary and page19).

CUTTING DOWN ON SODIUM

The amount of sodium (salt) we consume varies greatly from person to person. People who eat mainly processed foods have the highest sodium intake, while those who eat mainly unprocessed foods, such as fresh fruit and vegetables, have the lowest.

On average, we need about 1 g sodium (about half a teaspoon of salt) a day for our bodies to function efficiently. Ordinarily, however, we eat anywhere from 5-15 g salt a day – and about three-quarters of the sodium we consume comes from the salt we add to food during cooking or at the table.

Doctors may prescribe a low-sodium (low-salt) diet, usually for a limited time, for conditions such as high blood pressure, kidney diseases and in cases of water retention (oedema). Often, this takes the form of a 'no salt added' diet, which restricts the eating of certain processed or very highly salted foods. While a little salt may be used in preparing food, no extra salt may be added at the table.

Many people cannot imagine cooking without salt because they believe food without salt doesn't have any flavour, but it is possible to 're-educate' our taste buds, by *gradually* reducing the amount of added salt to allow our taste buds time to adapt to the lower levels. As a rule of thumb, if we avoid highly salted foods and remove the salt cellar from the table, we can reduce our sodium intake significantly!

These foods are high in sodium:
- Stock cubes or powder
- Baking powder, bicarbonate of soda and self-raising flour
- Flavoured salts such as celery, onion or garlic salt
- Commercial spreads, sauces and flavourings such as mayonnaise, prepared mustard, tomato sauce, horseradish sauce, Marmite, Bovril, Worcestershire sauce, braai sauce and soy sauce
- Salted and flavoured butter and salted spreads
- Prepacked herb and spice mixtures containing salt
- Canned meat and fish
- Smoked and processed meats such as ham, bacon,

salami, biltong, corned beef, frankfurters, luncheon meats, salt pork, sausage, smoked tongue
- Smoked and processed fish and seafood such as anchovies, caviar, salted herring, sardines, canned smoked mussels and oysters, smoked haddock, smoked salmon, fish pâté and spreads
- Hard cheese, especially Cheddar, Parmesan, Pecorino, Gouda and Havarti
- Soft cheese, especially processed cheeses, ricotta, mozzarella, Brie, Camembert and savoury cottage cheese
- Olives, pickles and salad dressings
- Instant foods, gravies and sauces
- Breakfast cereals
- Savoury breads, biscuits and crackers
- Salty snacks such as potato crisps, salted nuts, salted popcorn, olives and pickles
- Canned, frozen or instant soups, bouillon and noodles
- Ready-made convenience foods, such as lasagne or pizzas
- Chinese meals (which may contain monosodium glutamate).

A **reduced-sodium diet** focuses on foods to be avoided altogether, foods that are restricted and foods that may be taken in moderation.

Foods to avoid:
- Ordinary and flavoured salts
- Prepared sauces and condiments (including curry mixes); monosodium glutamate; baking powder and bicarbonate of soda
- Instant and quick-cooking hot cereals; commercial bread products made from self-raising flour or mealie meal; salted snacks
- Pickles, including olives; dried tomatoes or peppadews; sauerkraut; vegetable juice
- Maraschino cherries; crystallised or glazed fruit; dried fruit preserved with sodium sulphate
- Buttermilk; chocolate milk; instant milk mixes; standard hard and soft cheeses; ready-prepared pudding mixes; commercial ice cream, sorbet and frozen desserts
- Cured, canned, salted or smoked meat, poultry and fish; canned fish; salted textured vegetable protein; peanut butter; salted nuts
- Salted chicken and bacon fat; commercial salad dressings; gravy; mayonnaise
- Canned or instant soup and bouillon.

Restricted foods (1-2 portions a day; see Dietary guidelines for healthy people, page 10)
- Standard breads; cooked cereals
- Fresh vegetables, and those frozen or canned *without salt*, such as artichokes, beetroot, carrots, turnips, celery, kale, Swiss chard
- Vegetables canned or frozen *with salt*, such as frozen mealies, lima beans, peas, mixed vegetables
- Standard low-fat milk and yoghurt
- Fresh and frozen meat, poultry and fish; low-sodium canned meat and fish; low-sodium peanut butter; unsalted cheese and cottage cheese
- Eggs
- Standard butter and margarine.

Foods allowed in moderation (3-4 portions a day; see Dietary guidelines for healthy people, page 10)
- Low-sodium breads, bread products and cereals; puffed rice; puffed wheat; pasta; rice
- Fresh, unsalted frozen or unsalted canned vegetables, excluding those restricted above
- Fruit and fruit juices
- Unsalted butter, margarine and nuts; low-sodium salad dressings and mayonnaise; olive and vegetable oils
- Herb and spice mixtures without added salt
- Soups, casseroles and dishes made with allowed foods and ingredients.

STRATEGIES TO CUT SALT INTAKE
- Add little or no salt at the table.
- Read the labels on bought products and avoid those listing salt or sodium in the ingredients.
- See also low-sodium cooking below.

LOW-SODIUM COOKING
- Cook without, or with only small quantities of, added salt.
- Use less water, and cook for shorter periods, to preserve the natural flavour of foods. Steaming or stir-frying are excellent cooking methods.
- Use yeast as a raising agent whenever possible, rather than baking powder, which contains high levels of sodium.
- Oil and flavoured oils add flavour, use for cooking or to flavour salad dressings and sauces.
- Vinegar, especially balsamic vinegar, and/or lemon

juice add flavour to sauces, meat dishes and vegetables. Add grated orange or lemon zest to sauces for meat and for puddings.

- Prepare foods with sodium-free flavorants such as fresh or dried herbs, spices, garlic, chives, ginger and lemon.

For example, use basil, oregano and marjoram in salads, casseroles and Italian dishes. Mint is delectable in salads, couscous or tabbouleh, and dill and caraway add flavour to cabbage, cauliflower and potatoes. Thyme, rosemary, sage and bay leaves are excellent in meat and fish dishes, and fennel goes extremely well with fish. Try sage with pasta, and coriander in all sorts of dishes. Cumin, turmeric, saffron and mustard seeds

GLOSSARY

Angina: A painful feeling of pressure or a 'stiff' feeling in and around the heart, with pain that can spread to the back, neck and arms. It is caused by a lack of oxygen to a part of the heart muscle.

Arteriosclerosis, the most common cause of cardiovascular diseases, is a condition characterised by plaque (fatty matter that forms in, and on, the walls of the blood vessels) and by loss of elasticity in the blood vessels. The common name for the condition is 'calcification (or hardening) of the arteries'.

Atherosclerosis is a degenerative disease of the arteries characterised by patchy thickening of the inner lining of arterial walls, caused by fatty deposits; a form of arteriosclerosis.

Cholesterol is produced in the body by the liver, and also occurs in foods such as liver and egg yolk. Some cholesterol, in combination with other fats and protein, leaves the liver via the arteries and goes to the body tissues. This cholesterol is called lipoprotein. The cholesterol that accumulates in the arteries is made from small particles of saturated fat in the blood. The cholesterol in food is not the only factor in raising blood cholesterol levels; total fat intake from food, as well as the cholesterol in the body and the intake of saturated fats, are also responsible.

Coronary disease (CD): Damage to the heart muscle as the result of the cessation of, or obstruction to, the flow of blood to the heart.

Electrolytes are salts that dissolve in water, which play a major role in maintaining the water balance in the body.

Fatty acids: Organic compounds consisting of a chain of carbon atoms with hydrogen attached and an acid group at one end. The essential fatty acids are needed for our bodies to absorb fat-soluble vitamins such as vitamins A, D and E.

Heart attack: Sudden tissue death, caused by blockages of blood vessels that feed the heart muscle.

Hydrogenated fats: Hardened vegetable oils that have lost their polyunsaturated character and the health benefits that go with it.

Hypertension (high blood pressure): Chronic elevated blood pressure.

Monounsaturated fats: Fats containing a fatty acid that is unsaturated at one point; for example, olive oil.

Omega-6 and omega-3 fatty acids: Polyunsaturated fatty acids recognised as important in human nutrition. Linoleic acid is an omega-6 fatty acid found in the seeds of plants and in the oils produced from them. Any diet that contains vegetable oils, seeds, nuts and whole-grain foods provides enough linoleic acid to meet our bodies' needs. Linolenic acid is an omega-3 fatty acid, that also includes EPA (eicosapentoic acid) and DHA (docosahexanoic acid), which are found in fish oils. These oils are essential for normal growth and development and they may also play an important role in the prevention of heart disease, hypertension and cancer. Darker-fleshed fish; for example, mackerel, pilchards and tuna, have a high omega-3 fatty acid content.

Osteoporosis – meaning, literally, porous bones – is a condition in which the density of bones is reduced. Osteoporosis is discussed fully on page 19.

Polyunsaturated fats: Fats which contain fatty acids having two or more points of unsaturation; for example, vegetable oils, soft margarine.

Saturated fats contain fatty acids that have no points of unsaturation.

Stroke: A stroke occurs when blood flow to a part of the brain is cut off. Also called cerebrovascular accident or cerebral thrombosis.

Thrombosis: A thrombus or blood clot may obstruct a blood vessel causing thrombosis, which results in gradual tissue death.

Coronary thrombosis occurs when blood flow is blocked in an artery that feeds the heart.

Total fat intake: A combination of all the fats in a person's daily diet (eating plan).

Triglycerides: The chief form of fat in the diet, and the main form of fat storage in the body.

Unsaturated fats contain fatty acids with one or more points of unsaturation; for example, monounsaturated and polyunsaturated fats.

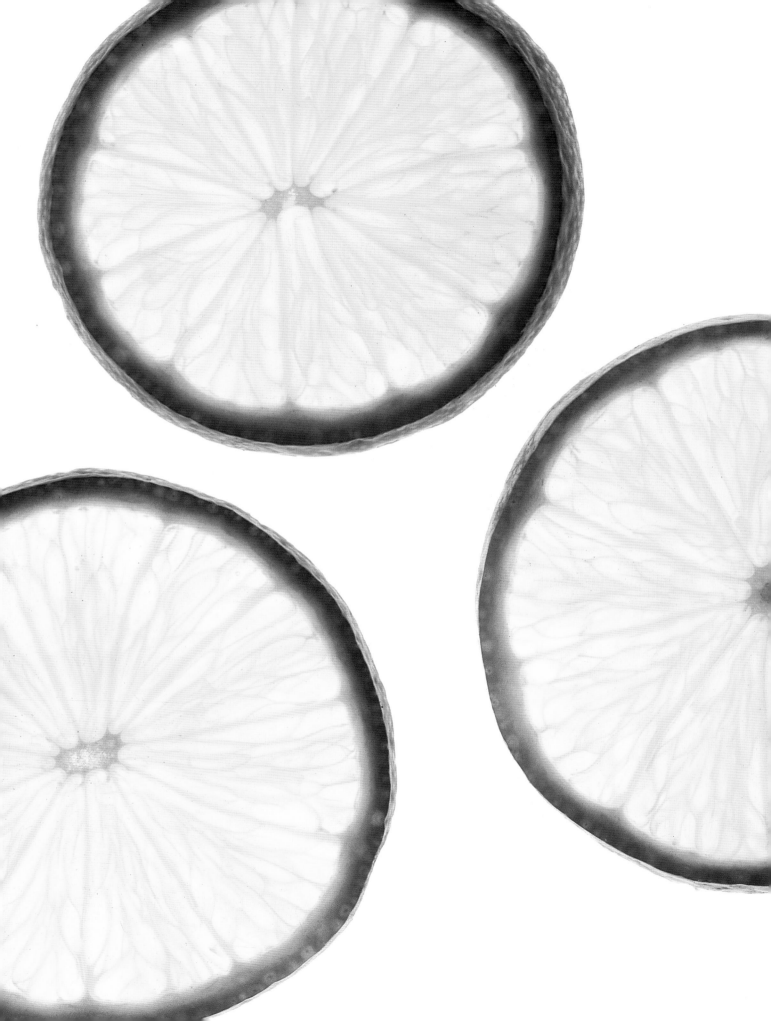

can be used to flavour lamb and mince dishes, and black, pink and green <u>peppercorns</u> add lots of flavour to all kinds of dishes. <u>Ginger</u>, <u>cinnamon</u> and <u>cloves</u> work well in stews and fish curries, as well as being excellent in breads, biscuits and desserts. <u>Chillies</u>, <u>paprika</u> and <u>coriander</u> disguise lightly salted dishes very well.

- Brown unsalted nuts and seeds lightly in an ungreased frying pan and sprinkle over dishes to add interest and flavour.

EATING OUT ON A REDUCED-SODIUM DIET

Restaurants may be accommodating, if you phone to warn them in advance. Other than this, the following tips will help:

- If you're ordering à la carte, or dishes prepared individually, you can ask that no salt be added.
- Order food without gravies, dressings or sauces.
- Steer clear of pasta dishes, soups or bouillon.
- Avoid Chinese food, which is traditionally very high in sodium.
- Choose fresh vegetables, salads and fruits where possible.
- Ask for olive oil and vinegar dressing on the side, so you can add as much as you want to your salad.

Fat is a more concentrated energy source than any other energy or macronutrient: 1 g fat yields 37 kJ (kilojoules); 1 g protein and 1 g carbohydrate each yields 17 kJ.

Diseases of the liver and gall bladder

The liver is the metabolic crossroads of our bodies, where, for example, carbohydrates, proteins and fat are metabolised; minerals and vitamins are stored and activated; and bile is formed. The liver is our bodies' detoxifier, and detoxifies, for example, alcohol. It's the only internal organ which, except under extreme disease conditions, can regenerate itself.

Two major diseases, hepatitis and cirrhosis, can cause permanent liver damage.

HEPATITIS

Hepatitis caused by HVA (hepatitis virus A), if treated timeously, will cause little or no permanent liver damage. The other strains are more virulent and might cause permanent liver cell destruction, leading to cirrhosis. Jaundice is the symptom of hepatitis, and is characterised by a yellowing of the skin, whites of the eyes and body fluids, resulting from the accumulation of bile pigments in the blood. Symptoms include fatigue, nausea, joint and muscle pain, loss of appetite, vomiting, diarrhoea and fever.

It is extremely important to diagnose hepatitis as soon as possible, in order to start treatment and prevent permanent liver damage.

TREATING HEPATITIS

Liver cells need all the nutrients to help them recover from hepatitis.

Here are some guidelines for treating hepatitis:

- Cut out all alcohol.
- Follow a well-balanced eating plan (see Dietary guidelines for healthy people, page 10), high in kilojoules and protein.
- Although it shouldn't be necessary to omit fat entirely from your diet, how much fat you can eat depends on your individual tolerance. If eating high-fat foods makes you feel nauseous, *stop*. If fat is not being absorbed properly, as is often the case in liver disease, you will have to follow a low-fat diet (page 49).
- Carbohydrates should provide about 55 percent of your energy needs; for example, if your kilojoule allowance is 10 000 kJ, at least 300 g of carbohydrates should be allowed. Include foods such as breads, vegetables and fruit.
- Eating small meals, often, is extremely important. Taking nutritional supplements may also help.
- Getting adequate rest is very important.

CIRRHOSIS OF THE LIVER

In this serious, chronic form of liver disease, liver cells are damaged to the point where they cannot regenerate and scar tissue forms, replacing liver cells that have permanently lost their function. Chronic alcohol abuse is one of the most common causes.

Because other conditions often accompany cirrhosis, treatment has to be individual, and your doctor will prescribe the regimen that's right for you.

GALLSTONES

The gall bladder produces bile, which is needed for fat metabolism.

'Gallstone disease' is the term given to the chronic formation of gallstones – which consist primarily of cholesterol, bilirubin and calcium salts – in the gall bladder. It's a fairly common condition and, in most cases, has no symptoms. The stones do, however, have the potential for serious complications. If they become lodged in the bile duct, for example, they could cause a painful obstruction and, if left untreated, can lead to pancreatitis, an inflammatory disease of the pancreas.

There's no specific dietary treatment to prevent gallstones forming. If the attack is severe, however, don't eat until the pain subsides, then follow a low-fat diet (see below).

LOW-FAT DIET

The low-fat diet allows about 40 g fat per day. Consult the list alongside for the daily allowances, as well as the list of foods allowed and not allowed to find out which fats you can choose from.

The following list outlines what is allowed and what you should avoid on a low-fat diet:

Drinks

Allowed: Skimmed milk; buttermilk made from skimmed milk; coffee; tea; fruit juice; soft drinks; cocoa made with cocoa powder and skimmed milk

Avoid: Full-fat milk; buttermilk made from full-fat milk; chocolate; cream (more than that allowed for under *fats*, below)

Bread and cereals

Allowed: Plain, fat-free cereals; pasta such as spaghetti, noodles, macaroni; rice; whole-grain or enriched bread; air-popped popcorn; bagels; English muffins

Avoid: Biscuits; breads other than whole-grain or enriched breads containing egg or cheese; sweet rolls made with fat; pancakes; doughnuts; waffles; fritters; popcorn prepared with fat; muffins; natural cereals and breads to which extra fat has been added

Cheese

Allowed: Cottage cheese (65 ml [¼ cup] to be used as a substitute for 30 g cheese), or low-fat cheeses containing less than 5 percent butterfat

Avoid: Full-fat cheeses

Desserts

Allowed: Sorbet made with skimmed milk; fat-free

FOOD	QUANTITY	APPROX FAT CONTENT (G) A DAY
skimmed milk	500 ml (2 cups) or more	0
lean meat, fish, poultry	180 g in total	18
whole egg or egg yolks	3 per week	2
vegetables	3 or more servings, with 1 or more dark green or deep yellow vegetables	0
fruit	3 or more servings, at least 1 citrus	0
breads, cereals as desired (fat-free)		0
fats and oil	4-5 tsp daily (= 5 g fat)	20-25
desserts & sweets	as desired, from list below	0
TOTAL FAT		38-43

frozen yoghurt; fruit ices; gelatine, rice, bread, cornflour or tapioca puddings made with skimmed milk; fruit whips with gelatine, sugar and egg white; fruit, angel food cake; digestive biscuits; vanilla wafers; meringues

Avoid: Cakes; pies; ice cream; any dessert containing shortening, chocolate, or fats of any kind, *unless specially prepared using part of fat allowance (see overleaf)*

Eggs

Allowed: 3 per week, prepared with fat from fat allowance (see below); egg whites as desired; low-fat egg substitutes

Avoid: More than 1 egg per day, *unless substituted for part of allowed lean meat*

Fats

Choose, to the limit listed, from the following (1 serving as listed = 1 fat choice): 5 ml (1 tsp) butter or margarine; 15 ml (1 tbsp) reduced-fat margarine; 5 ml (1 tsp) shortening or oil; 5 ml (1 tsp) mayonnaise; 10 ml (2 tsp) Italian or French dressing; 15 ml (1 tbsp) reduced-oil salad dressing; 1 rasher bacon, crisply fried; ⅛ small avocado; 30 ml (2 tbsp) light cream; 15 ml (1 tbsp) thick cream; 6 small nuts; 5 small olives

Avoid: All other fats, including those in excess of the quantities listed above

Fruit

Allowed: All

Avoid: Avocado in excess of quantity allowed for above

Lean meat, fish, poultry and meat substitutes

Allowed: Choose, up to the limit listed, from poultry without skin; fish; veal (all cuts); liver; lean beef, pork and lamb (all visible fat removed) – 30 g cooked weight = 1 choice; water-packed tuna or salmon – 65 ml (¼ cup) = 1 choice; tofu or tempeh – 90 g = 1 choice

Avoid: Fried or fatty meat; sausage; frankfurters; poultry skin; stewing steak; spare ribs; salted pork; beef (unless lean); duck; goose; ham hocks; pig's feet; luncheon meats; gravies (unless fat-free); tuna and salmon packed in oil; peanut butter

Milk

Allowed: Skimmed milk; buttermilk or yoghurt made from skimmed milk

Avoid: Full-fat, 2%, 1%, milk; chocolate milk; buttermilk made from full-fat milk

Seasonings

All allowed

Soup

Allowed: Bouillon; clear broth; fat-free vegetable soup; cream soup made with skimmed milk; packaged dehydrated soups

Avoid: All other soups

Diabetes mellitus

The word 'diabetes' comes from the Greek word for 'siphoning' or 'passing through', and the term refers to the large quantity of urine, with a high glucose (sugar) content, passed by people who have the disease. 'Mellitus' comes from the Greek word for 'honey'. Diabetes is often also referred to as 'sugar sickness' or 'sugar diabetes'.

The term actually describes a group of disorders, all characterised by abnormally high quantities of glucose in the blood, which is excreted in the urine due to the malfunctioning of the system that controls the amount of sugar in the blood.

HOW OUR BODIES CONVERT GLUCOSE INTO ENERGY

A certain quantity of **glucose** (see Glossary) in the blood is normal, and indeed necessary to supply energy to the entire body. When the glucose doesn't metabolise properly, the level remains high and is then secreted in the urine. Certain complications may arise, however, and the condition is then known as diabetes mellitus.

Insulin (see Glossary) is a hormone that enables our body cells to absorb glucose from the blood and store it (as glycogen) in the muscles and liver for later use, when energy is needed. Insulin is produced in the pancreas, a small gland that lies behind the stomach, which also produces digestive juices to help with the digestion of food.

After food has been digested, absorbed and glucose has been produced, the quantity of glucose in our blood increases. The pancreas then releases the correct quantity of insulin to transport the extra glucose to the cells, and the quantity of glucose in the blood returns to normal. When too little, or no, insulin is produced, or if the cells cannot absorb the insulin, diabetes develops.

TYPES OF DIABETES

There are two major types of diabetes:
- Type 1 diabetes, previously known as Insulin-dependent Diabetes mellitus (IDDM); and
- Type 2 diabetes, until recently called Non-insulin-dependent Diabetes mellitus (NIDDM).

Another two types of diabetes also occur:

- Gestational diabetes, which may occur during pregnancy; and
- diabetes that results as a complication from other conditions, such as diseases of the pancreas, or from certain medication.

TYPE 1 DIABETES

This is the less common of the two major types, and occurs when the pancreas cannot produce insulin. It's estimated that about 10 percent of South Africans who suffer from diabetes have Type 1. Our bodies' energy metabolism is drastically altered when there is no insulin available and the consequences are so severe that people with Type 1 diabetes cannot survive unless they have regular insulin injections.

Although Type 1 diabetes can develop at any age, it's more commonly diagnosed in children and adolescents. The exact cause is unknown, but it is thought that one cause might be a virus, which leads to the destruction of the part of the pancreas that manufactures insulin.

Because there is no insulin, the high levels of blood glucose cannot reach body cells; and because the glucose is unavailable, the body burns up its fat stores – too quickly to obtain energy. This will eventually result in a coma; a condition known as ketosis.

If you have some of the following symptoms, your doctor may diagnose Type 1 diabetes: **hyperglycaemia** (see Glossary) or high blood glucose levels, dehydration, drowsiness and glycosuria (glucose in the urine), which result in excessive urination and extreme thirst and hunger. You may lose a lot of weight in a short time, even though you have a large appetite. Your vision may be blurred, and you may also be extremely tired.

The treatment for this type of diabetes is insulin injections and a special diet. Insulin must be injected as your digestive juices will destroy it if you take it by mouth. Injected insulin is not broken down by your body, so you shouldn't miss meals if you're on insulin medication.

TYPE 2 DIABETES

This is the most common type of diabetes worldwide, which results from insufficient insulin production by the pancreas, and/or resistance to its action.

Type 2 diabetes develops slowly and symptoms are often less severe than in Type 1 diabetes. It usually develops in people over the age of 40, and the only symptom might be a high blood glucose level.

A number of factors may influence the development of Type 2 diabetes: a family history of diabetes; overweight and obesity; age; high blood pressure; stress; and lack of exercise.

Typically, the pancreas produces some insulin, but not enough. A high body weight or excess body fat complicates matters because it restricts the action of the insulin in carrying glucose to the cells (often referred to as insulin resistance).

Treatment for this type of diabetes includes following a healthy diet (see Dietary guidelines for healthy people, page 10), plenty of exercise and losing weight. If these measures aren't enough, medication to stimulate insulin secretion, or insulin injections, may have to be given. Even with well-controlled diabetes, it may be necessary to give extra insulin or oral medication during periods of illness or emotional stress, or after surgery.

GESTATIONAL DIABETES

As the term suggests, this type of diabetes develops during pregnancy. It is found in about 5,5–8 percent of all pregnancies, and is caused by the increased levels of some hormones that decrease the effectiveness of insulin action.

Although this type of diabetes disappears with the birth of the baby, about half of the women who suffer from gestational diabetes will develop Type 2 diabetes within 20 years. Women who experience this type of diabetes during their pregnancy should, therefore, control their weight, exercise regularly and follow a healthy diet in order to minimise the risk factors.

IMPAIRED GLUCOSE TOLERANCE

This is the body's inability to regulate its blood glucose concentration adequately in response to the intake of glucose or carbohydrates, or the release of glucose from body cells during fasting or times of metabolic stress (which can be trauma resulting from illness, or emotional stress). These people have blood glucose levels above the normal range, but not so high as to be diagnosed with diabetes. Following a healthy eating pattern, taking regular exercise and long-term weight control will make a big

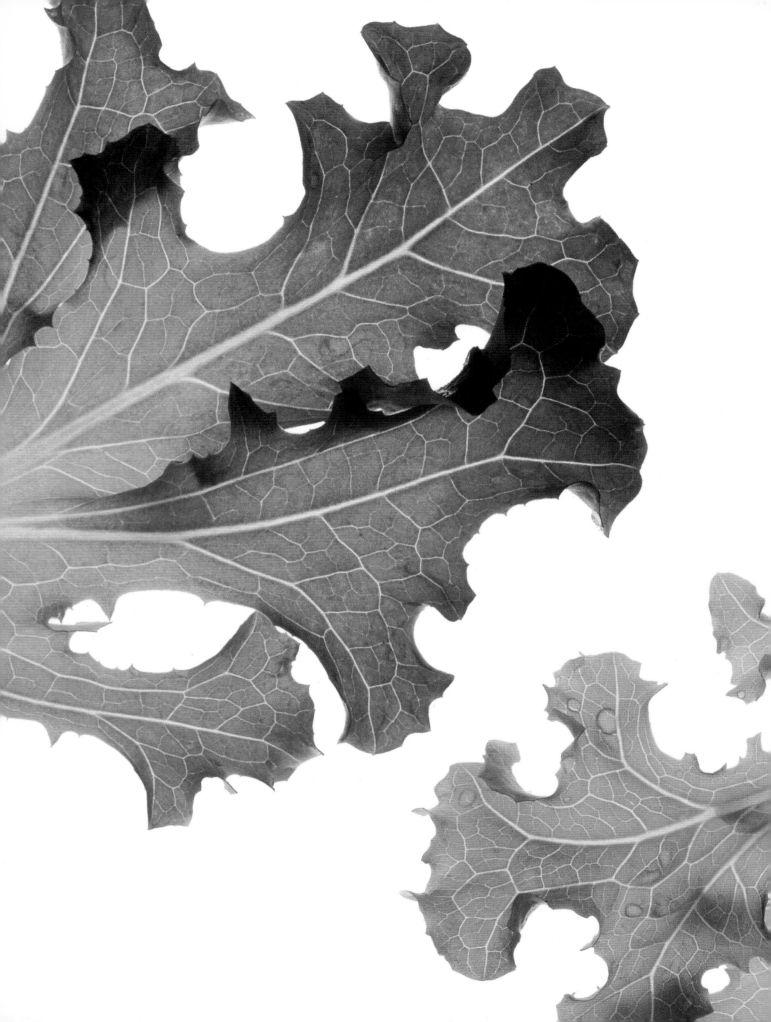

difference. Of people following this regimen, a third will improve, a third will remain glucose-intolerant and a third will develop Type 2 diabetes.

DIAGNOSING DIABETES
Diagnosis is made by taking a blood test. This can be a fasting blood glucose test, taken when you have been without any food or drink (except water) for 10 to 12 hours; a random test, which can be taken at any time; or a postprandial test, taken 2 hours after eating.

BLOOD GLUCOSE LEVELS*		
	Fasting	After a meal
Optimal	4–6	5–8
Acceptable	6–8	8–10

* Measured in mmol/litre

If the results are not clear, you may be given a glucose tolerance test. You will have to fast for 10 hours, after which you will be given 75 g liquid glucose to drink. Your blood sugar level is then measured at set intervals.

Another blood test is the Glycosylated haemoglobin level (HBA1c), which shows the level of glucose in the blood over the past two months.

COMPLICATIONS OF DIABETES
Complications may be acute (immediate) or chronic (over a longer period).

Acute complications are:
- High blood glucose (sugar) levels, or hyperglycaemia, and sugar in the urine
- Ketosis or coma
- Weight loss (Type 1 diabetes)
- Weight gain (Type 2 diabetes)
- **Hypoglycaemia** (see Glossary) or low blood glucose levels, which may be the result of poor management of diabetes, especially in Type 1, where insulin is given.

Chronic complications: If a diabetic's blood glucose levels remain high or fluctuate excessively over a period, it may damage the blood vessels supplying the eyes, kidneys, heart and other organs, as well as the nerves, especially in the legs and feet. Infections are more likely because of poor circulation coupled with the glucose-rich blood and urine. Cardiovascular diseases tend to develop and progress more rapidly in diabetics.

MANAGING DIABETES
The treatment goals are to:
- Maintain blood glucose levels within a fairly normal range
- Achieve optimal blood lipid (fat) levels
- Control blood pressure levels
- Prevent complications as far as possible, and treat them if necessary
- Support health and wellbeing.

Exactly which approach is the most beneficial for you will depend on what type of diabetes you have, your weight, age and level of fitness.

Monitoring your blood glucose levels every day will help you get to know your body and how to control your diabetes. It will give you an idea of the effect of food, exercise and medication on blood glucose levels.

To ensure that you control diabetes as you should, you should visit your doctor, dietician or other health-care professional regularly.

THE DIABETIC'S DIET
If you have Type 1 diabetes, your doctor will prescribe insulin and an eating plan to match. Type 2 diabetics should follow a healthy eating plan (see Dietary guidelines for healthy people, page 10). It's important, however, to pay attention to *all* the nutrients that provide energy. Controlling the type and quantity of carbohydrates you consume will prevent hyperglycaemia and hypoglycaemia; controlling your protein intake and the type and quantity of fats you eat will help prevent cardiovascular complications.

CARBOHYDRATES, SIMPLE AND COMPLEX SUGARS AND THE GLYCAEMIC INDEX
To control blood glucose levels, the diabetic needs to have glucose available all day long. Once eaten, carbohydrates – both starches and sugars – will raise blood glucose levels in about an hour.

Complex carbohydrates such as whole-grain bread and cereals, legumes, fruit and vegetables are preferable to simple sugars, such as sweets, cakes, sugar and honey because they also provide fibre, vitamins and minerals. Concentrated sweets may be eaten as a limited part of a healthy diet, provided that diabetics count them as part of their carbohydrate allowance.

Different carbohydrate foods (sugars and starches) have different effects on blood glucose levels, even when they provide the same quantity of carbohydrates. Some cause a quicker, higher rise in blood glucose levels than others, because their digestion and/or absorption rates are different.

The Glycaemic Index (GI) rates foods from 1 to 100, according to the effect they have on blood glucose levels. Foods that are digested and absorbed slowly cause a small rise in blood glucose levels and have a low GI value, whereas foods that cause a greater rise have a higher number. To control diabetes, it is better to concentrate on foods with a low GI value, provided that they are also low in fat.

Processing, preparation and cooking, the quantity and type of fibre and the quantity of fat all affect a food's GI value.

The more a food is *prepared*, the easier it is for your body to break it down and absorb the carbohydrate. Smooth-textured whole-wheat bread, for instance, will have a higher GI value than coarser, heavier whole-wheat bread.

The more a food is peeled, chopped and cooked, the easier it is for your body to absorb the carbohydrate. Stewed fruit, for instance, is easier and quicker to absorb than fresh fruit.

Glucose is absorbed quickly and therefore has a high GI number, whereas fructose (fruit sugar) is absorbed slowly and has a low GI number. Sucrose (cane sugar) comes somewhere in between and has a medium GI number. Unfortunately, all these sugars have the same kilojoule content!

Fibre, especially bran and oats, slows down the digestion and absorption of carbohydrates and therefore reduces the GI value.

Because fat slows down digestion, high-fat foods will also have a low GI value. But fat also causes overweight and can cause heart disease. For this reason, diabetics should keep their intake of fats to the minimum.

Include low-GI foods regularly in your eating plan, to help control and even out swings in blood glucose levels. But remember that individual responses to foods vary.

CUTTING DOWN ON SUGAR

Here are some hints for cutting down on your sugar intake:

- Check the labels on products on the supermarket shelves and avoid those that use terms such as dextrose, disaccharides, honey, grape concentrate, lactose, malt, malt extracts, maltose, mannitol, sorbitol, molasses, sucrose, treacle, xylitol, brown sugar, invert sugar. And remember: 'no sugar added' does not necessarily mean the product doesn't contain sugar from other ingredients, as in fruit juices.
- Don't add sugar to drinks and cereals.
- Drink water rather than fruit juices and other sweetened drinks.
- Choose products canned in water or in unsweetened fruit juice rather than syrup.
- Low-fat fruit yoghurt is sometimes very high in sugar, so read the label carefully.
- Use less sugar than a recipe states; adding fruit or fruit juices instead of sugar or syrup will often provide enough sweetness.
- Don't add sugar to vegetables; they often have enough natural sweetness of their own.
- Train your palate to prefer less sugar, but if you really cannot do without, use artificial sweeteners (see Artificial sweeteners, page 55).

ALCOHOL AND THE DIABETIC

Alcoholic drinks are high in kilojoules (about 30 kJ to a gram), and they're readily absorbed by the body.

A standard drink would be 30 ml spirits such as whisky, gin, brandy or vodka; 60 ml sherry, vermouth or port; 120 ml wine; and 200 ml beer.

Bear in mind that sweeter wines contain more sugar, and remember to add in the amount of sugar in mixers such as lemonade and cola drinks. All liqueurs contain a lot of sugar and are high in kilojoules.

Here are a few tips:

- So-called 'diabetic' beers and wines are often high in alcohol, so check the alcohol content on the label.
- Mix wine with ice-cold water or soda water to make it last longer. Drinking plenty of water along with alcoholic drinks is also a good idea.

- Never drink an alcoholic drink on an empty stomach because it will be absorbed into the blood stream immediately.
- Eating starchy foods with drinks will also slow down the absorption of alcohol.

IMPORTANT: If you're on medication for hyperglycaemia, or taking insulin, and you drink alcohol without taking some carbohydrate food, it may react with the medication and cause a substantial drop in blood glucose levels.

A SHORT GUIDE TO SWEETENERS

Sweeteners that do not supply kilojoules

- Acesulphane-K (marketed as Sucaryl™ and Assugrin Gold™) contains aspartame and is about 200 times sweeter than sugar. It is used in a wide variety of manufactured food products, such as soft drinks, yoghurt or fruit drinks. It can leave a bitter aftertaste, but is not metabolised by the body.
- Aspartame is marketed under a variety of trade names, such as Canderel, Equal and so on. It can be used in many recipes in place of sugar, but because it tends to break down under high heat or when cooked for a long time, it should rather be added at the end of the cooking process. It leaves no aftertaste and is 180 times sweeter than sugar.
- Cyclamate was banned in the USA and the UK when it was found that a very high intake might cause liver and/or kidney damage in laboratory animals. It is, however, still widely used elsewhere in the world. In South Africa, cyclamate is often used, especially in soft drinks. Natreen™, a liquid sweetener, is a combination of cyclamate, saccharin and Acesulphane-K. The Carcinogen Assessment Group in the USA has determined that cyclamate does not cause cancer in humans.
- Saccharin is 300 times sweeter than sugar but a bitter or metallic aftertaste is a problem for many people. To curb this effect, add it as late as possible in the cooking process. It is marketed in South Africa as Sweetex™ and Hermesetas™.

Sweeteners that supply kilojoules

- Sorbitol is manufactured commercially from glucose obtained from fruit. It is absorbed slowly into the blood and, although it will not cause a major increase in blood glucose levels, it will supply kilojoules. In large quantities, it has a laxative effect.
- Mannitol contributes about half the quantity of kilojoules of sugar because it is poorly absorbed. It is also less sweet than sugar.
- Fructose occurs naturally in fruit and honey. It contains the same quantity of energy (kJ) per weight as glucose but is absorbed slowly and has a low GI value. It needs less insulin to metabolise than sugar and can be used sparingly by diabetics.

ARTIFICIAL SWEETENERS

Using artificial sweeteners in drinks and cooking will help to control the quantity of sugar you take in and, consequently, maintain a normal range in your blood glucose level.

There has been some controversy about the safety of artificial sweeteners, but the concerns have so far not proved positive.

COOKING WITH ARTIFICIAL SWEETENERS

Here are some hints:

- Read the label on the sweetener to find out what its kilojoule (kJ) count is. Some products marketed as 'sugar free' in fact contain fructose or sorbitol, which adds kilojoules.
- If a sweetener leaves a bitter or metallic aftertaste, experiment with different ones or a combination of sweeteners.
- Cyclamate and saccharin are ideal for dishes such as crème brûlée, which are not cooked to high temperatures. Cyclamate and saccharin tend to become bitter when boiled, particularly with fruit, so add after cooking.
- Aspartame loses its sweetness when heated, making it unsuitable for cooking. It also loses its sweetness with prolonged storage.

EATING AT HOME

Regular meals will help to control blood sugar levels, and when you're on diabetes medication, it's very important to be punctual about meal times.

Having diabetes doesn't affect your need for energy and nutrients – carbohydrates, proteins, fats, minerals and vitamins – *but it does affect the timing and planning of meals*. Changing your eating pattern may be difficult, so it may be better to change the timing and dose of medication instead; but consult your doctor or dietician first.

Ensuring that you eat at least a few carbohydrate food portions at every meal will help to spread the carbohydrates in such a way that it will keep your blood glucose levels within an acceptable range. And, depending on your medication, a carbohydrate-rich snack between meals may be recommended.

EATING OUT
Having diabetes doesn't mean a lifetime of deprivation and missing out on the fun, but you should know about diabetes and its complications if you are to make common-sense choices when eating out:
- Read the menu carefully or have a good look at a buffet table. In most cases, you can ask that sauces and gravies be left out altogether, or have them served on the side.
- Vegetables and salads are always available.
- A plain grilled portion of meat or fish with a baked or boiled potato and extra bread are all good choices.
- Most dessert menus feature fruit; otherwise you can have a starter and skip dessert.
- When eating out at someone's home, your hostess won't be affronted if you leave certain foods you cannot eat on your plate.
- Limit your alcohol intake and ask for water on the side.

TRAVELLING
Always take whole-wheat crackers, fruit and water with you, so you can be sure you have carbohydrates available in case you have a hypoglycaemic incident. If you're travelling by air, you can order special meals when you make your booking. If you're going to be crossing time zones, discuss this with your doctor beforehand so that you can sort out your insulin and food requirements.

EXERCISE AND DIABETES
Exercising is a very important part of the overall treatment plan for diabetes because it helps keep blood glucose levels within the normal range. It will also help to keep your body weight normal.

If you have Type 2 diabetes you can actually cut out

or reduce the need for medication if you regularly exercise or take part in sport.

If you have Type 1 diabetes, it's important to know your body and to be aware of the signs of hypoglycaemia and hyperglycaemia. Where possible, check your blood glucose level before exercising, especially if you have recently been diagnosed. Always carry high-carbohydrate snacks with you: sweets, soft drinks, dried fruit and biscuits, for instance. After vigorous exercise, your blood sugar level will continue to drop for some time, so have a snack afterwards. Guard against dehydration, and keep drinking plenty of liquids. Alcohol isn't a good idea, however, as it may lower your blood glucose level even more.

DIABETES AND PREGNANCY
Well-managed diabetes isn't a problem if you're pregnant, although it is important to have good medical supervision and to adjust insulin doses and meal plans.

DIABETES AND CHILDREN
A diagnosis of diabetes mellitus in a child or teenager is often a shock, and guilt feelings, as well as resistance and anger, sometimes surface. This is perfectly normal. The way to handle it is to gain knowledge about the disorder, and not to panic.

It's important for your child to take an active part in managing his or her diabetes, as well as in diet planning and general monitoring; for example, of blood glucose levels. What sometimes helps is to provide a role model – perhaps a sports star, or a pop singer – who also has diabetes, so that your child doesn't feel alone. The SA Diabetes Association (head office: 011-788-4595/6, or consult your local telephone directory for a branch near you) has information about camps and other activities which double as training sessions for diabetes management.

Here are some tips for coping with your child's diabetes:
- Avoid making diabetes the focal point of your household; it will single out your child and cause other siblings to rebel.
- Plan for sweets and desserts in your child's diet; you may find that if you deny them, your child will see them as something to binge on, or to eat surreptitiously.

- Guard against being manipulated. Children very soon learn to manipulate situations, and you could find that your child will refuse certain foods in the hope of getting snacks.
- Make sure that friends, and their parents, as well as teachers – especially the sports trainer – know the basics of your child's diet.
- Always give your child sweets and/or extra snacks to take with him or her, so that a hypoglycaemic incident can be treated, should it occur.

Remember that hormonal changes and growth spurts during adolescence may upset diabetes control. You may find that you have to adjust and reassess your child's management routine.

WHAT TO DO IF SOMEONE DISPLAYS THE SYMPTOMS OF HYPOGLYCAEMIA

- IF THE PERSON IS *UNCONSCIOUS*, GET MEDICAL HELP STRAIGHT AWAY.
- IF THE PERSON *BECOMES UNCONSCIOUS*, ROLL HIM OR HER ONTO HIS OR HER LEFT SIDE AND CLEAR THE MOUTH OR AIRWAYS OF FOOD. CALL MEDICAL HELP IMMEDIATELY.
- IF THE PERSON IS *NOT UNCONSCIOUS* AND IS ABLE TO SWALLOW:
- IMMEDIATELY GIVE HIM OR HER SOME SUGAR TO RAISE THE BLOOD GLUCOSE LEVEL. CHOOSE FROM:
  - 4–6 GLUCOSE-ENRICHED SWEETS OR JELLY BEANS
  - 1 GLASS GLUCOSE-ENRICHED DRINK (BUT NOT LOW-KILOJOULE OR ARTIFICIALLY SWEETENED DRINKS)
  - 30 ML (2 TBSP) JAM OR HONEY
- IF SYMPTOMS PERSIST AFTER 5 MINUTES, ADMINISTER MORE SUGAR, AS ABOVE. IF THERE'S STILL NO IMPROVEMENT AFTER 10 MINUTES, CALL A DOCTOR OR GO TO THE EMERGENCY DEPARTMENT OF YOUR LOCAL HOSPITAL WITHOUT DELAY.
- ONCE SYMPTOMS DISAPPEAR, ADD A SNACK CONTAINING MORE COMPLEX CARBOHYDRATES, SUCH AS WHOLE-WHEAT BREAD OR PASTA. DON'T INCLUDE ANY OF THE ABOVE IN THE USUAL MEAL AND TREATMENT PLAN.

GLOSSARY

Glucose: A monosaccharide (single) sugar that is a major energy source in the body's metabolism.

Hyperglycaemia: High blood glucose levels. The symptoms are: Intense thirst and (sometimes) hunger; increased urination; blurred vision; acetone-smelling breath; glycosuria (glucose in the urine) and laboured breathing.

Hypoglycaemia: Low levels of glucose in the blood; one of the complications of diabetes. The symptoms are: hunger, headaches, sweating, shakiness, nervousness, confusion, disorientation and slurred speech. A blood glucose level of below 3,5 mmol should be treated as hypoglycaemia.

Possible reasons for hypoglycaemia are: taking too much insulin (previously known as insulin shock); a delayed meal; too little carbohydrate in the food to match the insulin; taking alcohol without eating some carbohydrate; unplanned activity, without carbohydrates to stabilise the blood sugar level; and stomach upsets, diarrhoea or vomiting. Left untreated, hypoglycaemia can lead to loss of consciousness, brain damage and even death.

CAUTION: Many of the symptoms of hypoglycaemia are the same as for alcohol intoxication. To ensure that the right diagnosis is made in an emergency, every person who suffers from diabetes should wear a Medic-Alert bracelet or necklace.

Insulin is a hormone secreted by the pancreas that enables our body cells to absorb glucose from the blood and store it in the muscles and liver for later use, when energy is needed. Your physician will prescribe the type, or combination, of insulin you will need, depending on your medical history and lifestyle.

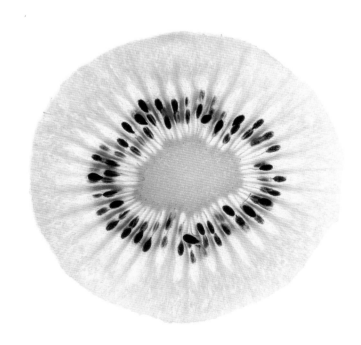

Nutrition and cancer

Cancer patients who are on antitumour therapy often experience unpleasant side effects. Special dietary guidelines, and avoiding certain foods, can help counteract some of them. The following are some of the side effects, and the nutritional treatments that might help:

SYMPTOMS: ACUTE GASTROINTESTINAL TOXICITY, NAUSEA AND VOMITING

Diet: Clear, cold, nonacidic liquids; light, low-fat foods
Avoid: Acidic liquids such as citrus, vinegar and alcohol; milk products; cream soups; fried foods; sandwiches; sweet desserts

SYMPTOMS: STOMATITIS (see Glossary), OESOPHAGITIS (see Glossary)

Diet: Liquid diet (page 37) and soft diet (page 38), such as broth-based soups, fruit drinks, carbonated drinks, melons; as well as changing the texture and temperature of foods to make them more acceptable and so avoid irritation
Avoid: Juices, especially citrus; bananas; crisp or raw foods; meat; spicy foods; textured or granular foods; coarse breads; extremely hot or cold foods
Supplements and aids: Mild-flavoured nutritional supplements; brush teeth often with nonirritating toothpaste; rinse mouth with a weak salt and water solution

SYMPTOMS: DRY MOUTH, PRODUCTION OF MUCUS

Diet: Soft, nonirritating diet; tea with lemon; fruit drinks; carbonated drinks; broth-based soups; thinned warm cereal
Avoid: Thick fruit nectars and other thick liquids; thick cream soups; thick hot cereals; breads; gelatine; oily foods
Supplements and aids: Artificial saliva (available from pharmacies); wash mouth often with a weak salt and water solution

SYMPTOM: DECREASED SALIVA PRODUCTION

Diet: Well-balanced diet (see Dietary guidelines for healthy people, page 10) of high-moisture foods such as gravies, sauces, casseroles, chicken, fish, sorbet, melons, vegetables with sauces; foods containing citric acid, such as citrus sweets; citrus fruits. Drink liquids with food

Avoid: Dry foods; breads; meat; crackers; bananas; excessively hot food; alcohol
Supplements and aids: Artificial saliva; saliva stimulants, such as sugarless lemon drops and gum; frequent saline rinses

SYMPTOM: MOUTH 'BLINDNESS' (see Glossary)

Diet: Well-balanced diet (see Dietary guidelines for healthy people, page 10) concentrating on strongly flavoured foods; emphasis on aroma and texture
Avoid: Bland foods, plain meat, unsalted foods
Supplements and aids: Flavoured nutritional supplements; wash mouth often with a weak salt and water solution

SYMPTOM: ALTERATIONS IN TASTE

Diet: Well-balanced diet (see Dietary guidelines for healthy people, page 10) containing many cold foods; milk products; emphasis on experimentation with foods
Avoid: Red meat; chocolate; coffee; tea
Supplements and aids: Fruit-flavoured nutritional supplements

SYMPTOM: EARLY SATIETY (QUICKLY FEELING FULL)

Diet: High-energy diet with the emphasis on kilojoule-dense foods such as meat, fish, poultry, eggs, full-cream milk, cheese, cream-based soups, ice cream, full-cream yoghurt, creamed vegetables, rich desserts; eat small meals, frequently
Avoid: Low-fat or fat-free milk products; broth-based soups; green salads; steamed plain vegetables; low-kilojoule drinks
Supplements and aids: Energy-dense supplements such as vitamins and minerals

SYMPTOM: CONSTIPATION

Diet: Well-balanced diet (see Dietary guidelines for healthy people, page 10) with extra fibre; extra fluids
Avoid: Foods and drinks that cause flatulence (see page 39)
Supplements and aids: Fibre-enriched nutritional supplements; bulking agents (available from pharmacies)

SYMPTOM: LOWERED RESISTANCE (see Glossary)

Diet: Safe-food diet – well-cooked foods with emphasis on cleanliness, because chemotherapy tends to cause the white blood cell count to drop and the patient is more prone to infections

Avoid: Raw fish; meat; mould-containing unpasteurised cheeses; tempeh; all miso products; raw, unpeeled fruit and vegetables; dried fruit; raw or fresh-roasted nuts; brewers' yeast; unpasteurised honey; commercial cream-filled pastries requiring refrigeration; dried and fresh spices added after cooking; herbal supplements

Supplements and aids: Wash hands often to keep them clean and avoid contamination; make sure food is handled safely.

NUTRITION AND AIDS

Patients receiving treatment for Aids often experience the same side effects as those receiving treatment for cancer. Follow the regimen for specific side effects listed here.

GLOSSARY

Mouth 'blindness': Loss of taste.

Lowered resistance: This can lead to being prone to infection.

Oesophagitis: Inflammation of the gullet.

Stomatitis: Inflammation of the mouth and corners of the mouth.

healthy living

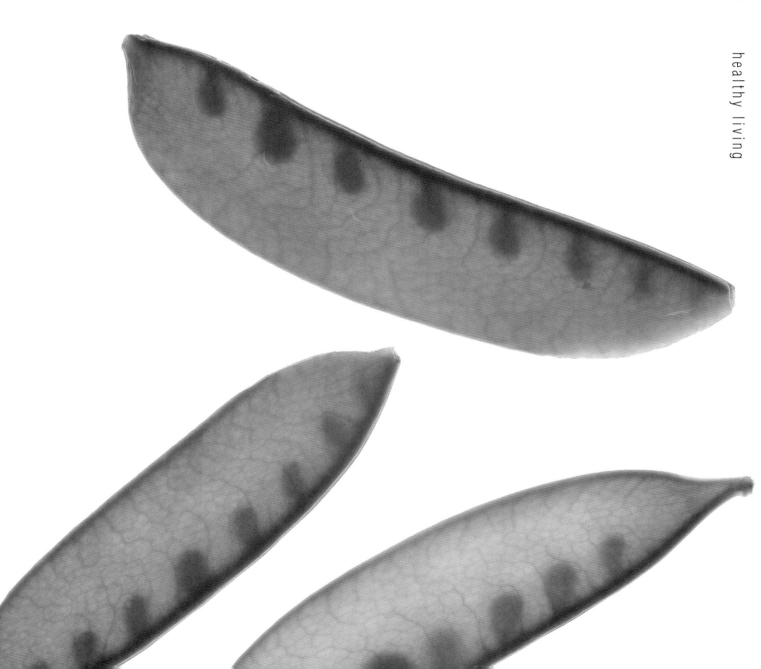

rec

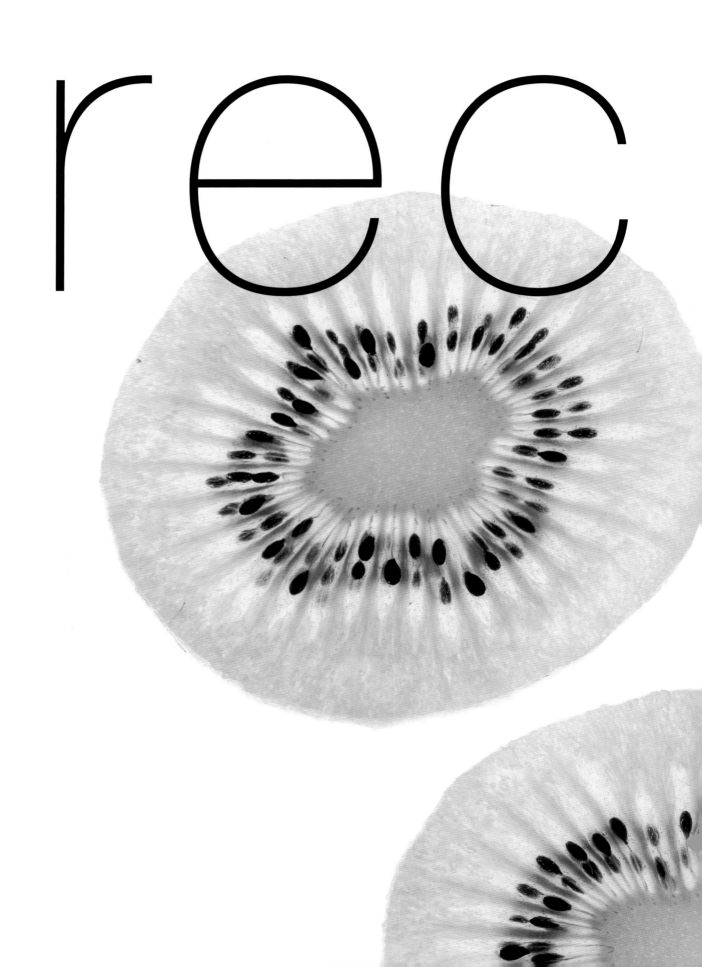

pes

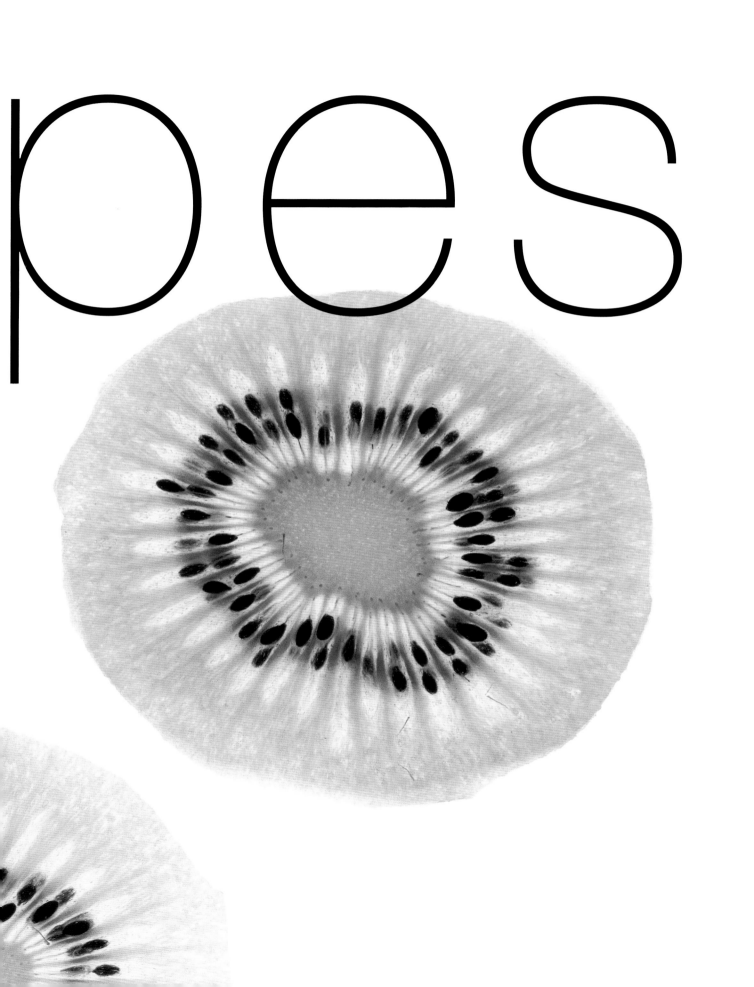

All the recipes have been chosen with a healthy lifestyle in mind – which means that they conform to the dietary guidelines outlined on page 10. Preference has been given to recipes that are lower in fat and sodium, higher in fibre and packed with essential nutrients.

We've also tried to provide variations and alternatives wherever possible, in the belief that eye and taste appeal are just as essential as the best possible combination of nutrients for attaining and maintaining healthy eating habits. Consequently, fresh fruit and vegetables are almost always called for, and only stand-bys such as pancakes and tortillas ever see the freezer. Remember: the fresher the fruit or vegetable, the higher its nutrient value will be.

INGREDIENTS

Wherever possible, the healthier alternative has been chosen. So, for example,

- low-fat natural yoghurt is preferred to fruit yoghurt or cream
- canola oil is recommended (though you can use whichever vegetable oil you prefer) because of its high percentage of polyunsaturated fats
- low-fat (or 2%) milk is generally preferred to fat-free or skimmed, although where milk powder is called for, skimmed milk powder is recommended
- high-sodium products such as soy sauce or Worcestershire sauce are either omitted or the quantity required is considerably reduced
- the quantity of sugar called for has been cut dramatically, or omitted altogether (and recipes have been chosen that do not use a lot of sugar); in some cases, fructose or other sugars may be used instead (for more information, see page 55)
- meat cuts have been chosen that contain less fat, such as lamb (not mutton), or where the fat can easily be removed, such as pork
- chicken breast fillets are almost always called for rather than chicken portions, because all the fat has already been removed.

PORTION SIZES

Portion sizes for the individual recipes were calculated in accordance with dietary guidelines for healthy people on page 10.

COOKING METHODS

To attain and maintain healthy eating habits, it is a good idea to use cooking methods that require little or no extra fat or oil, such as dry-pan grilling (for meat and fish), stir-frying, grilling, baking, poaching and steaming. We have avoided using fat-and-oil-based cooking methods, such as deep-frying, pot-roasting and roasting (except where the food being roasted contains little fat and only the minimum quantity of oil or cooking fat has been added).

WEIGHT MANAGEMENT

While we have not annotated appropriate recipes as being helpful in losing or maintaining weight, we have assigned a kilojoule value to every recipe, which will enable you to calculate whether it fits in with your daily kilojoule allowance.

Remember, too, that the kilojoule values given are approximate, and rounded off to the nearest 5; so do not use them in calculations where an exact value is required.

SPECIAL DIETS

The emphasis, as we have stated before, is on nutrient-rich dishes that reduce the quantities of, or eliminate, the fats, sugar and salt called for, or offer alternatives to foods that cannot be eaten by people with special dietary needs.

Where applicable, we have given, with each recipe, an indication of the kind of diet for which the recipe is suitable. You will find this information at the end of the recipe, at a heading that reads *Suitable for*. When we refer here to 'low fat', 'low gluten', 'low cholesterol', etc., we are referring to the kind of diet. If you are in any doubt about whether a recipe is suitable, consult your dietician.

- *Diabetics* should, as always, ensure that they adhere to their daily eating plans and allowances, and use discretion when choosing recipes to try.
- Those who have a *gluten intolerance* should look for recipes that are indicated as 'low gluten'.
- If you have to watch your *fat or cholesterol intake*, look for recipes that are termed suitable for 'low fat' and 'low cholesterol'.

MEASURES

We have used metric measures throughout. For convenience, here are the conversions for cups, teaspoons and tablespoons:

1 ml = ¼ teaspoon
2 ml = ½ teaspoon
5 ml = 1 teaspoon
10 ml = 2 teaspoons
15 ml = 3 teaspoons OR 1 tablespoon

15 ml = 1 tablespoon
30 ml = 2 tablespoons
45 ml = 3 tablespoons
60 ml = 4 tablespoons
75 ml = 5 tablespoons
90 ml = 6 tablespoons

50 ml = ⅕ cup
65 ml = ¼ cup
85 ml = ⅓ cup
100 ml = ⅖ cup
125 ml = ½ cup
150 ml = ⅗ cup
170 ml = ⅔ cup
190 ml = ¾ cup
200 ml = ⅘ cup
250 ml = 1 cup
375 ml = 1½ cups
500 ml = 2 cups
750 ml = 3 cups
1 litre = 4 cups

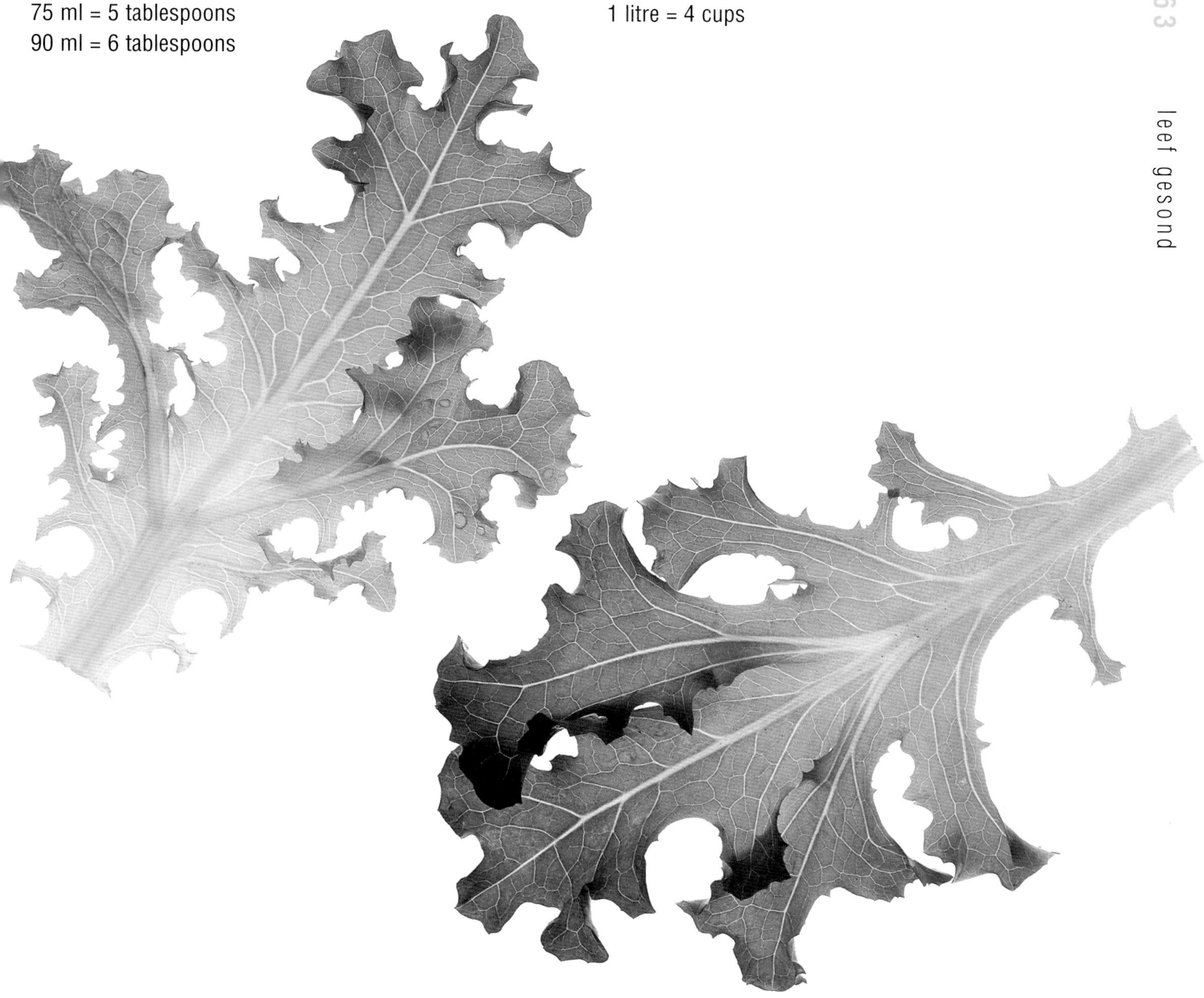

leef gesond

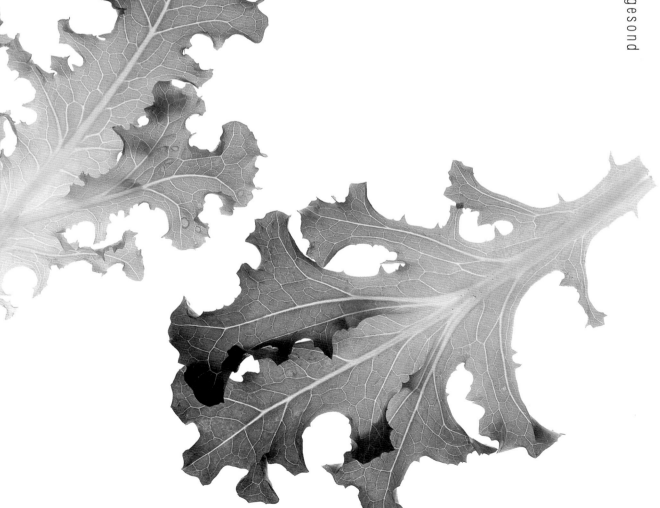

Starters and soups

The first course sets the tone for a meal, and stimulates the appetite for what is to follow. Our selection of nutritious, lower-fat appetisers and soups prove that it is possible to tantalise the taste buds without piling on the kilojoules!

HINT

WHEN MAKING SOUP, IT'S BETTER TO USE HOME-MADE STOCK, BECAUSE THAT WAY YOU CAN CONTROL HOW MUCH FAT AND SALT THE STOCK CONTAINS. SEE OUR RECIPE FOR LOW-SALT CHICKEN STOCK (PAGE 149), WHICH MAKES AN EXCELLENT BASE FOR SOUPS AND OTHER DISHES.

Snoek sambal

(Makes 375 ml)

Snoek sambal makes an excellent starter to a traditional meal.

500 g cooked snoek, skin and bones removed and flesh flaked
1 onion, peeled and finely chopped
2 ml chilli sauce or Tabasco sauce
10 ml vinegar
2 ml salt
2 ml pepper
5-10 ml moskonfyt or apricot jam

Mix all the ingredients together well and serve with thinly sliced whole-wheat bread and butter or with whole-wheat crispbread.
140 kJ per 15 ml serving

Suitable for: low gluten, low cholesterol.

Crudités with three dipping sauces

(Serves 4-6)

The three dips make this the perfect first course for a special dinner or lunch.

½ small head cauliflower or broccoli
4 carrots
2 red, green or yellow sweet peppers
2 celery stalks
10 cm piece English cucumber
1 baby gem or cos lettuce
6 large mushrooms

Steam the cauliflower or broccoli until crisp-tender, about 10 minutes, then cut into florets. Peel the carrots and cut into julienne strips. Core and seed the peppers, and cut into strips. Trim the celery and cut into fingers. Cut the cucumber into rounds and separate the lettuce into leaves. Wash and drain the carrots, peppers, celery, cucumber and lettuce (or whizz in a salad spinner). Wipe the mushrooms with a damp cloth and slice horizontally, stalks and all, into quarters. Chill the vegetables until ready to serve. Arrange the vegetables on platters and serve with all the dips, or with just one or two.
250 kJ per serving

● High in fibre.

Creamy dill dip

(Makes 300 ml)

50 ml chopped fresh dill or 10 ml dried
25 ml chopped fresh parsley
250 ml smooth cottage cheese or fromage fraîs
45 ml low-fat natural yoghurt
salt and freshly ground black pepper to taste

Chop the fresh dill and parsley in a food processor or blender. Add the cottage cheese and yoghurt and season to taste. Process, pulsing until the desired texture is achieved. Transfer to a bowl, cover and chill until ready to serve.
50 kJ per 15 ml serving

Spicy avocado dip
(Makes about 300 ml)

1 ripe avocado, peeled and stoned
45 ml low-fat natural yoghurt
pinch crushed dried chillies
5 ml freshly squeezed lemon juice
freshly ground black pepper to taste

Mash the avocado and stir in the remaining ingredients. Pack into a dish, cover and chill until ready to serve.
170 kJ per 15 ml serving

Coriander chicken dip
(Makes 350 ml)

200 ml chopped cooked chicken breast meat
¼ small red sweet pepper, cored, seeded and
sliced
50 ml reduced-oil mayonnaise
salt and freshly ground black pepper to taste
2 sprigs fresh coriander

Place the chicken and red pepper in a food processor or blender and chop coarsely. Add the mayonnaise, seasoning and coriander and chop again, to the desired texture. Transfer to a bowl, cover and chill until ready to serve.
230 kJ per 15 ml serving

● Use chicken breast fillets and poach in lightly s
ed water to which 1 bay leaf and 2 whole pepp
corns have been added.

Suitable for: low gluten, low cholesterol.

Marinated mushrooms
(Serves 4-6)

If Mediterranean is your thing, add strips of roasted and skinned red sweet pepper and a black olive or two

450 g small mushrooms
65 ml extra-virgin olive oil
30 ml lemon juice
1 clove garlic, halved
2 bay leaves
pinch dried oregano
2 ml salt
pinch freshly ground black pepper

Remove the stems from the mushrooms. Wipe the caps clean with a cloth or paper towel and place them in a container with a tight-fitting lid.
Combine the remaining ingredients in a saucepan and bring to the boil. Remove from the stove and allow to cool. Pour the mixture over the mushrooms in the container, cover and refrigerate for at least 2 days, shaking occasionally. To serve, pour off the marinade and place the mushrooms in a serving dish lined with lettuce leaves.
660 kJ per serving

Suitable for: low cholesterol.

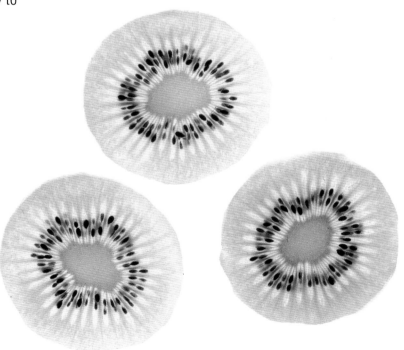

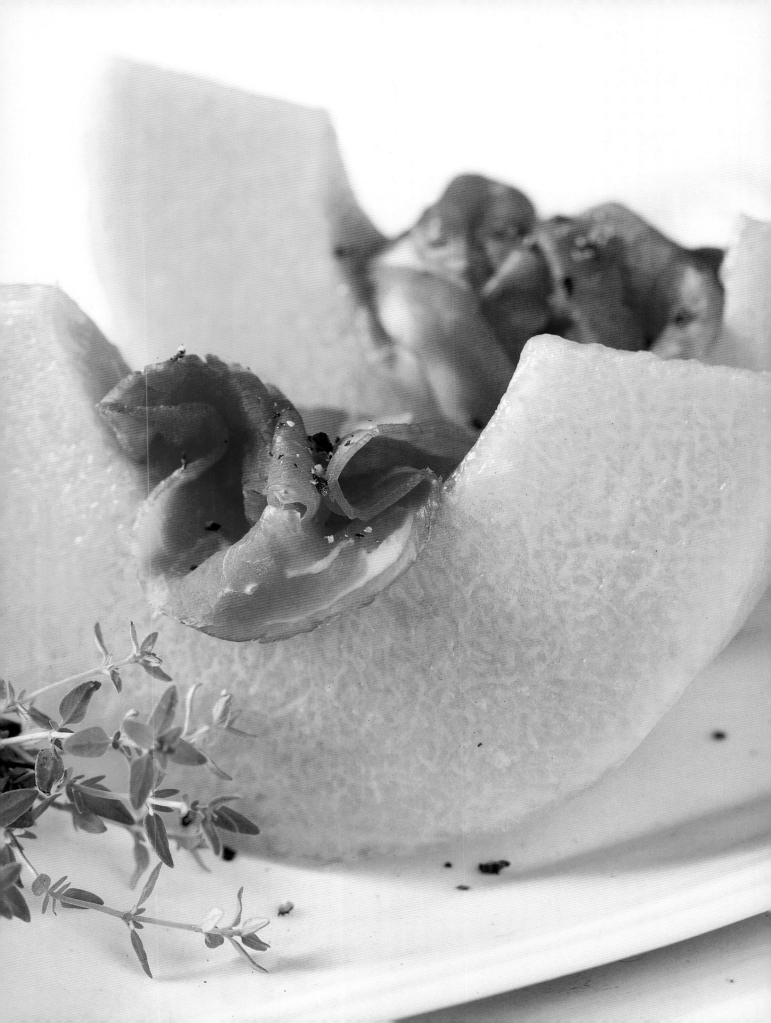

Sweet melon with shaved beef

(Serves 4-6)

This variation on the classic melon and Parma ham starter features an unusual combination of beef and melon.

1 medium spanspek, honeydew melon or Ogen melon, peeled, seeded and sliced
8-12 slices shaved beef
freshly ground black pepper

Arrange 2 slices of melon per person on plates, top with 2 slices of beef and grind a little black pepper over.
355 kJ per portion

VARIATION: USE SHAVED TURKEY, CHICKEN OR HAM INSTEAD OF SHAVED BEEF.

Suitable for: low gluten.

Brinjal pâté

(Makes about 250 ml)

Brinjals are also known as aubergines and eggplant. Whatever you call it, this is a delectable way to enjoy the vegetable. Brinjal pâté may be made up to a day in advance and stored, covered, in the refrigerator.

1 large brinjal
canola oil for brushing
1 slice white bread, crust removed
1 clove garlic, crushed
1 spring onion, finely chopped
15 ml finely chopped fresh parsley
5 ml chopped fresh marjoram
salt and freshly ground black pepper to taste
30 ml extra-virgin olive oil
fresh lemon juice

Preheat the oven to 190 °C.
Brush the brinjal skin with canola oil and bake for 40-60 minutes, or until soft. Set aside to cool. Halve the brinjal and scoop the flesh into a blender or food processor. Soak the bread in cold water, then squeeze it dry. Add to the brinjal with the garlic, spring onion, herbs, salt and pepper and purée until smooth. Gradually add the oil, beating constantly. Adjust the seasoning, if necessary, and add lemon juice to taste. Transfer to a bowl, cover and chill until needed. Serve with rosemary breadsticks (recipe on page 136).
150 kJ per 15 ml serving

VARIATION: SERVE AS PART OF THE CRUDITÉS PLATTER.

Suitable for: low cholesterol, low fat.

Falafel

(Serves 8)

Enjoy these Middle Eastern patties on their own, with a dip, or in pitta breads with salad ingredients.

450 g canned chickpeas
1 egg, lightly beaten
2 ml turmeric
30 ml chopped fresh coriander leaves or parsley
1 ml ground cumin seeds
1 ml cayenne pepper
1 clove garlic, crushed
15 ml tahini (sesame paste)
100 ml crushed wheat, soaked and drained
salt and freshly ground black pepper to taste
100 ml cake flour
canola oil for deep-frying

Combine the chickpeas, egg, turmeric, coriander or parsley, cumin, cayenne pepper, garlic, tahini and crushed wheat in a blender or food processor. Purée until smooth, then season to taste with salt and pepper. Shape the mixture into 2 cm diameter balls and flatten them slightly. Dust with flour and deep-fry in hot oil until lightly browned, about 5 minutes. Drain well on absorbent paper and serve hot.
750 kJ per serving

- Tahini is available from some supermarkets (look on the health food shelves) and from health stores.
- High in fibre.

Hummus

(Makes about 500 ml)

Hummus may be prepared a few hours in advance and chilled until needed.

400 g cooked chickpeas
100 ml water
2 cloves garlic, crushed
150 ml tahini (sesame paste)
juice of 1 lemon
7 ml salt
freshly ground black pepper to taste
pinch ground cumin
pinch chilli powder
chopped fresh coriander leaves to garnish

Purée the chickpeas and water in a blender or food processor. Gradually beat in the garlic, tahini and lemon juice to taste. The mixture should spread easily – add a little more water if it is very thick. Season to taste with salt and pepper, cumin and chilli powder and garnish with coriander leaves. Serve with breadsticks or crudités.
680 kJ per 15 ml serving

- Tahini is available from some supermarkets and from health stores.
- This dish is fibre-rich.

VARIATION: USE 1 X 410 G CAN CHICKPEAS AND MAKE THE CANNING LIQUID UP TO 100 ML WITH WATER.

Suitable for: low gluten, low sodium (omit salt).

Asparagus with red pepper purée

(Serves 6)

Make this only if you can get fresh asparagus – the red peppers bring out their delicate flavour.

2 large sweet red peppers
10 ml olive oil

1 ml dried thyme
freshly ground black pepper
1 kg fresh asparagus spears

Preheat the oven to 190 °C.
Place the peppers on a baking sheet and roast for 18-20 minutes. Turn and roast the other side for 18-20 minutes, or until the peppers are blistered and soft. Remove from the oven and place in a plastic bag. Close the bag and let the peppers steam for 10-15 minutes. Using a small knife and your fingers, peel off the skin from the peppers, remove the seeds and cores and cut the flesh into strips. Heat the oil over moderate heat. Add the peppers and thyme and sauté for 2 minutes. Season with pepper to taste, then purée in a food processor or blender.
Wash the asparagus and break off the tough ends. Steam in a large saucepan of boiling water for 5-8 minutes, or until tender. Drain thoroughly.
Spoon the hot pepper purée over individual plates and arrange the hot asparagus on top.
235 kJ per serving

Suitable for: low gluten, low sodium.

Chilled soups

Using really fresh vegetables is particularly important when soups are to be served chilled, as their flavour is much more prominent. Serve the soups in chilled bowls for best results.

Gazpacho

(Serves 6)

This is the classic chilled tomato soup, which originated in Spain. Although fresh tomatoes are best, you can also use 2 x 400 g cans of peeled Italian tomatoes, and their juices.

1 kg fresh ripe tomatoes, peeled and coarsely chopped
1 small cucumber, peeled and finely chopped
½ onion, peeled and finely chopped

1 stalk celery, trimmed and finely chopped
1 clove garlic, crushed
25 ml tomato purée
125 ml cold water
50 ml olive oil
25 ml white wine vinegar
2 slices white bread, crusts discarded
10 ml salt
freshly ground black pepper to taste

TO SERVE
chopped cucumber
chopped tomato
chopped onion or spring onion
black olives
chopped chives and parsley

Place all the ingredients in a blender or food processor and purée until smooth and thick. Chill for 2 hours before serving with all, or a few of, the listed vegetables and herbs.
600 kJ per serving

Suitable for: low cholesterol, low fat.

Chilled yoghurt and cucumber soup
(Serves 4)

A ridge cucumber can be used, but English cucumbers have a better flavour.

1 medium-sized English cucumber
500 ml low-fat natural yoghurt
10 ml freshly squeezed lemon juice
5 ml olive oil
5 ml finely chopped fresh mint leaves
2 ml finely chopped fresh dill
5 ml salt

Peel the cucumber, slice it lengthways, then scoop out and discard the seeds. Grate the cucumber coarsely. In a deep bowl, stir the yoghurt with a whisk until it is completely smooth. Gently whisk in the grated cucumber and all the other ingredients. Chill the soup for at least 1 hour and serve in chilled soup bowls.
400 kJ per serving

CHILLED CUCUMBER AND CHIVE SOUP: USE LOW-FAT BUTTERMILK INSTEAD OF YOGHURT, AND CHIVES AND PARSLEY INSTEAD OF MINT AND DILL.

Suitable for: low fat, low cholesterol, low gluten.

Chilled carrot and coriander soup
(Serves 6)

The soup may also be served hot, accompanied by Melba toast or whole-wheat bread or rolls.

1 onion, peeled and chopped
500 g young carrots, scraped and sliced
5 ml ground coriander
875 ml chicken stock or low-salt chicken stock
  (recipe on page 149)
50 ml chopped fresh coriander leaves
salt and freshly ground pepper
natural yoghurt, sunflower seeds, coriander
  leaves or parsley sprigs to garnish

Combine the onion, carrots, coriander and chicken stock in a saucepan and simmer, covered, until the vegetables are tender, 15-20 minutes. Purée the mixture until smooth. Stir in the fresh coriander and seasoning to taste. Chill. Serve in chilled bowls, garnishing each serving with a spoonful of yoghurt, a sprinkling of sunflower seeds and chopped fresh coriander or parsley.
245 kJ per serving

● High in fibre.

To cook in the microwave: Combine the onion, carrots, ground coriander and 25 ml chicken stock in a microwave-safe dish. Cover and microwave on 100% power for 8-12 minutes, or until carrots are tender. Continue as described in the recipe.

Suitable for: low fat, low cholesterol.

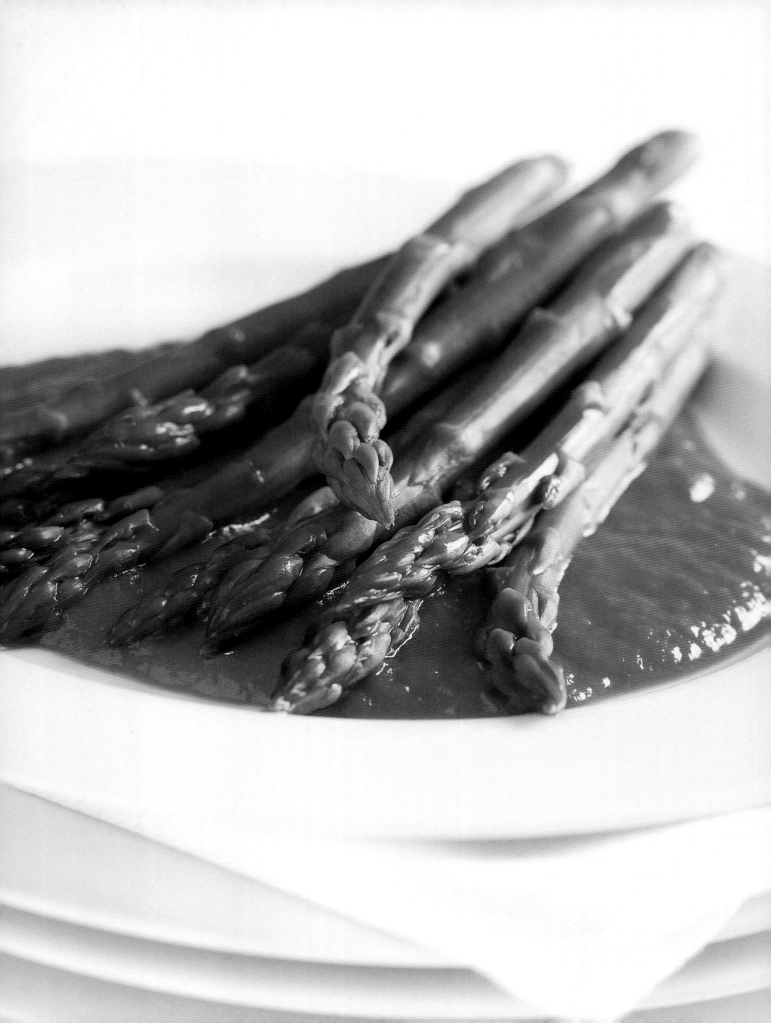

Chilled petits pois soup

(Serves 4)

This soup has a beautiful pale green colour, and a delectably light flavour to match. Serve in a glass serving dish, standing in crushed ice, for greater eye appeal.

250 g frozen petits pois
25 ml medium cream sherry (optional)
175 ml low-fat natural yoghurt
250 ml cold chicken stock or low-salt chicken stock (recipe on page 149)
2 ml onion juice (optional)
freshly ground black pepper to taste
mint sprigs to garnish

Thaw the peas slightly and place in a blender or food processor with the sherry (if using). Purée until smooth. Add the yoghurt, stock and onion juice (if using) and mix lightly. Season to taste with black pepper. Transfer to a serving dish and chill well. Serve garnished with fresh mint.
600 kJ per serving

Suitable for: low cholesterol.

Hot soups

Beat the cold with warming soups, filling enough to be a one-pot supper. Although packed with flavour, the soups given here are not high in kilojoules, fat or salt, which makes them perfect for those wishing to lose weight, or who have to watch their fat and salt intake.

Chunky chicken and vegetable soup

(Serves 4)

A more interesting variation on chicken noodle soup, this soup also packs a lot more oomph.

1 litre chicken stock or low-salt chicken stock (recipe on page 149)
1 bouquet garni
2 chicken breast fillets
65 ml long-grain white rice, or brown rice
1 large carrot, peeled and cut into strips
1 stalk celery, trimmed and thinly sliced
250 ml sliced mushrooms
125 ml frozen peas
50 ml chopped fresh parsley
freshly ground black pepper to taste

Place the stock and bouquet garni in a saucepan, cover and bring to the boil, then reduce the heat to moderate. Add the chicken and rice and simmer until the chicken is cooked, about 10 minutes. Remove the chicken with a slotted spoon and transfer to a plate.
Simmer the soup until the rice is just tender, 10-15 minutes. Dice the chicken and return to the soup. Add the carrot, celery, mushrooms, peas and parsley, and remove the bouquet garni. Cook for 5 minutes, or until the vegetables are crisp-tender. Season with black pepper to taste, and serve with whole-wheat rolls.
470 kJ per serving

● High in fibre.

Suitable for: low fat, low cholesterol, low sodium (use low-salt stock).

Potato and leek soup

(Serves 4)

Smooth, velvety and simply delicious!

15 ml butter or canola margarine
3 large leeks, trimmed and chopped
1 small onion, peeled and chopped
450 g potatoes, peeled and chopped
1,25 litres chicken stock or low-salt chicken stock (recipe on page 149)
150 ml low-fat milk
freshly ground black pepper to taste
30 ml snipped fresh dill or chives to garnish

Melt the butter or margarine in a large saucepan. Sauté the leeks and onion until softened but not browned, about 10 minutes. Add the potatoes and stock. Bring to the boil and simmer for 15-20 minutes, or until the potatoes are tender. Purée until smooth, then return to the saucepan and add the milk. Season to taste with black pepper and reheat gently to just under boiling point. Serve garnished with the dill or chives.
820 kJ per serving

Suitable for: low cholesterol, low fat, low sodium (use low-salt stock).

Vegetable soup with mini-meatballs

(Serves 4-6)

The meatballs may be made up to 2 hours in advance and chilled until needed.

1 litre chicken or vegetable stock, or low-salt chicken stock (recipe on page 149)
4 medium carrots, peeled and cut into strips
250 ml frozen peas
½ head cauliflower or broccoli, broken into florets
2 potatoes, peeled and diced
250 g green beans, topped and tailed and sliced
1 leek, trimmed and sliced
5 ml chopped fresh mint to garnish

MEATBALLS
250 g extra-lean steak mince or ostrich mince
½ small onion, peeled and finely chopped
1 slice white bread, soaked in milk and the excess milk squeezed out
1 egg
5 ml chopped fresh parsley
2 ml salt
1 ml freshly ground black pepper
100 ml dried breadcrumbs

First make the meatballs. Combine all the ingredients except the breadcrumbs. Shape into small balls, roll in breadcrumbs and chill while making the soup.
Heat the stock in a large saucepan. Add the vegetables and cook for 15 minutes, then add the meatballs and cook for a further 10 minutes. Season, if necessary. Sprinkle with mint and serve.
320 kJ per serving

● High in fibre.

Suitable for: low fat, low cholesterol.

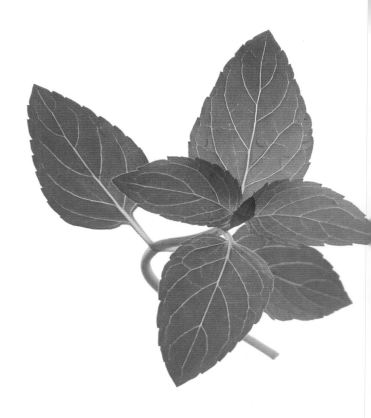

72

Lentil soup
(Serves 4)

Serve this flavourful soup on a cold day, and warm yourself from the inside out!

250 ml red or brown lentils
10 ml butter, margarine or canola oil
4 lean bacon rashers, chopped
1 small onion, peeled and finely chopped
1 small carrot, peeled and thinly sliced
1 celery stalk, trimmed and thinly sliced
1,5 litres chicken stock or meat stock, or low-salt
  chicken stock (recipe on page 149)
salt and pepper to taste
croutons to serve

Soak the lentils in water to cover for 30 minutes. Drain and pick over the lentils. Heat the butter, margarine or canola oil in a large saucepan. Add the bacon and stir-fry until cooked but not too crisp. Add the onion, carrot and celery and stir-fry for a few minutes. Add the chicken stock and lentils and bring to the boil, then reduce the heat and simmer, stirring occasionally, until the vegetables and lentils are tender, about 30 minutes. Purée the soup, season if necessary, then return the soup to the saucepan and heat through. Serve topped with croutons.
360 kJ per serving

● High in fibre.

Suitable for: low fat (omit bacon).

Fish chowder
(Serves 4)

Fish chowder makes a hearty, one-pot meal that's both satisfying and nutritious.

15 ml butter or canola oil
1 onion, peeled and finely chopped
3 potatoes, peeled and diced
1 carrot, peeled and finely chopped
500 ml water
500 ml low-fat milk
500 g white fish fillets, cut into chunks
250 ml whole-kernel corn
100 ml frozen petits pois or minted garden peas
salt to taste
pinch freshly ground black pepper
chopped fresh parsley

Melt the butter or canola oil in a heavy-based saucepan, add the onion, potatoes and carrot and cook over moderate heat, stirring occasionally, for 5 minutes. Add the water, cover and simmer until the vegetables are nearly tender, about 15 minutes.
Stir in the milk, fish, corn and peas. Simmer for 5-10 minutes or until the fish flakes easily and is opaque. Add salt, pepper and parsley to taste.
1 080 kJ per serving

● For low-fat diets, make the soup in a nonstick saucepan.

MUSSEL CHOWDER: USE COOKED MUSSEL MEAT IN-STEAD OF FISH FILLETS.
CORN CHOWDER: OMIT THE FISH. CHOP AND SAUTÉ 4 LEAN BACON RASHERS IN A SAUCEPAN UNTIL CRISP. CONTINUE WITH THE RECIPE, USING 1 X 425 G CAN CREAMSTYLE SWEETCORN INSTEAD OF WHOLE-KER-NEL CORN AND ADDING A FEW THIN STRIPS OF RED SWEET PEPPER.

Suitable for: low gluten, low cholesterol.

Salads

This selection of salads provides options for hot summer days, as well as more robust offerings for cooler evenings. Most vegetables are high in fibre, not to mention vitamins and minerals, so they are always a good choice.

Tzatziki

(Makes about 500 ml)

Icy cold, minty fresh, this is the ideal counterpoint to grilled lamb or pork.

1 English cucumber, peeled and finely diced
salt and freshly ground black pepper
2 cloves garlic, crushed
30 ml finely chopped fresh mint
250 ml low-fat natural yoghurt
15 ml fresh lemon juice
chopped fresh mint to garnish

Place the cucumber in a sieve, sprinkle with salt and leave to drain for 1 hour. Mix the remaining ingredients, except the garnish, seasoning to taste. Rinse the cucumber in cold water and combine with the yoghurt mixture. Serve garnished with chopped mint.
50 kJ per serving

Suitable for: low fat, low cholesterol.

Sousboontjies

(Serves 6)

A quick version of the traditional favourite.

200 g dried sugar beans
cold water
25 ml butter
25 ml sugar

25 ml water
50 ml vinegar
2 ml salt

Soak the beans overnight in cold water to cover. Drain, cover with fresh water and cook until the beans are tender. Drain, add remaining ingredients and simmer gently for 10 minutes. Serve hot or cold.
680 kJ per serving

● High in fibre.

Suitable for: low gluten.

Salad Caprese

(Serves 4)

It looks great and tastes even better! Add thinly sliced cucumber and pitted black olives, if you wish, to provide an authentic Mediterranean touch.

2 large ripe tomatoes, skinned and thickly sliced
8 thin slices mozzarella cheese, halved
125 ml chopped fresh basil or basil leaves

DRESSING
30 ml olive or canola oil
15 ml lemon juice or balsamic vinegar
salt and freshly ground black pepper
1 clove garlic, crushed

Arrange the tomato slices in overlapping circles on a flat serving dish. Arrange the mozzarella slices in a circle over them and sprinkle with basil.
Place the dressing ingredients in a screw-top jar and shake well to combine. Drizzle over salad just before serving.
385 kJ per serving

Suitable for: low gluten, low fat (use low-fat cheese), low cholesterol (use low-fat cheese).

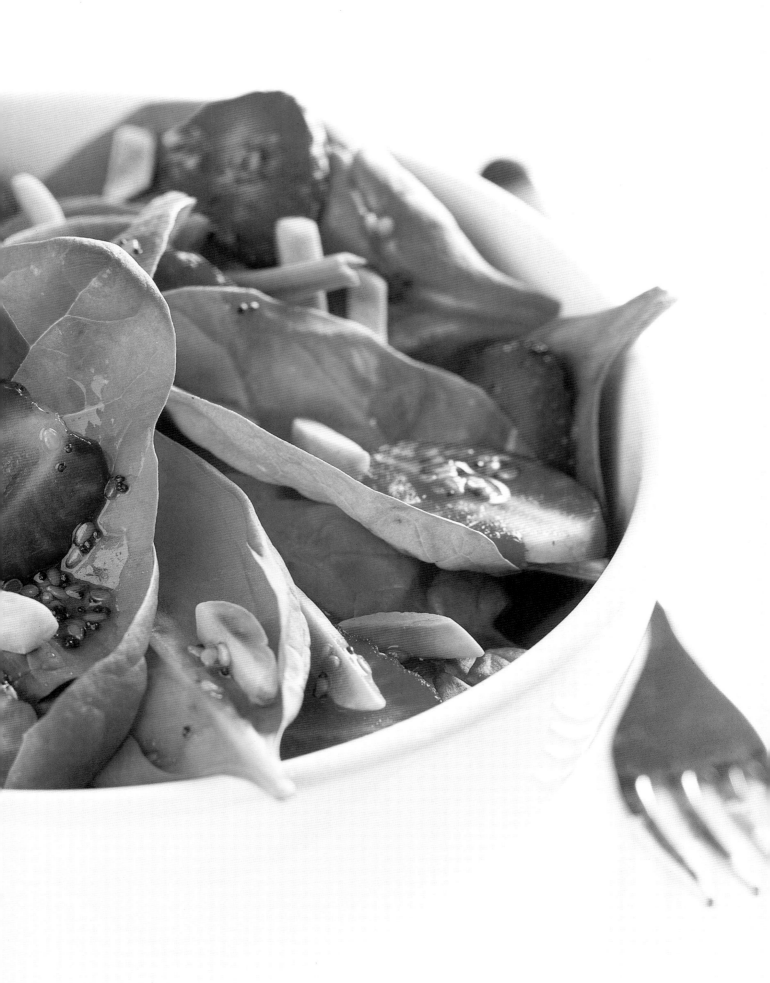

Spinach salad with sesame seed dressing

(Serves 10)

An excellent salad for the buffet table. The recipe may be halved.

500 g spinach
75 ml sliced almonds
500 ml firm strawberries, washed, hulled and sliced

DRESSING
15 ml sesame seeds
50 ml cider vinegar
45 ml walnut or canola oil
45 ml water
15 ml sugar
5 ml poppy seeds
1 ml paprika
1 ml Worcestershire sauce
1 spring onion, minced

Preheat the oven to 180 °C.
Trim, wash and dry the spinach and place in a salad bowl.
Sprinkle the almonds on a baking sheet and roast in the oven for 5 minutes, or until golden. Set aside.
To make the dressing, place the sesame seeds in an ungreased frying pan and stir over moderate heat until lightly browned. Combine the seeds, vinegar, oil, water, sugar, poppy seeds, paprika, Worcestershire sauce and spring onion in a bowl and mix well.
Just before serving, drizzle the dressing over the spinach and toss well to coat. Add the strawberries and almonds and toss lightly.
390 kJ per serving

VARIATION: INSTEAD OF USING ALMONDS AND STRAWBERRIES, ADD 6 BACON RASHERS, SLIVERED AND FRIED UNTIL CRISP, 50 ML PINE KERNELS AND ABOUT 8 OLIVES, STONED AND CUT INTO STRIPS. WOULD PUSH UP FAT CONTENT.

Suitable for: low gluten, low fat.

Sugar snap pea and tomato salad with strawberry vinaigrette

(Serves 4)

Fresh or frozen raspberries may be used instead of strawberries in the vinaigrette.

500 g sugar snap peas or mangetout, topped and tailed
250 ml bean sprouts
250 g Rosa tomatoes, halved

VINAIGRETTE
250 g strawberries
85 ml cider vinegar
250 ml extra-virgin olive oil
5 ml canned green peppercorns, drained
5 ml sugar
1 clove garlic, crushed
(Makes 625 ml)

Steam or microwave the sugar snap peas or mangetout until just tender, then drain. Rinse under cold water and drain again. Combine the peas in a bowl with the bean sprouts and tomatoes. Toss with strawberry vinaigrette just before serving.
To make the vinaigrette, blend or process all the ingredients together until smooth.
400 kJ per serving

● Store the vinaigrette in a jar in the refrigerator and use as a salad dressing for many salads.

● High in fibre.

Suitable for: low gluten, low cholesterol.

Bulgur

(Serves 8)

A crunchy, fibre-packed Middle Eastern salad that's becoming ever more popular throughout the world.

75 g crushed wheat
cold water
4 tomatoes, skinned and finely chopped
½ English cucumber, finely chopped
1 green sweet pepper, cored, seeded and finely chopped
½ medium onion, peeled and finely chopped
60 ml chopped fresh parsley
15 ml finely chopped fresh mint
juice of 2 lemons
60 ml olive oil
salt and freshly ground black pepper

Soak the crushed wheat in cold water to cover for 1 hour. Drain well, wrap in a clean dish towel and press out all excess moisture. Spread the wheat out on a tray to dry. Place the prepared vegetables in a mixing bowl with the dried crushed wheat. Stir in the parsley, mint, lemon juice and olive oil, season with salt and pepper and serve.
400 kJ per serving

● High in fibre.

Suitable for: low cholesterol, low fat.

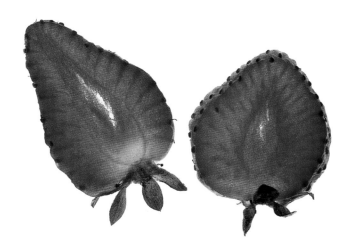

Green salad with apple dressing

(Serves 6-8)

The ingredients for the salad can vary, depending on what you have available. Little Gem lettuce is a good addition, and so are the frilly lettuces, celery, asparagus and crunchy green apples.

100 g watercress, trimmed
1 small oak-leaf lettuce, separated into leaves
1 small cos lettuce or red butter lettuce, separated into leaves
1 small butter lettuce, separated into leaves
10 young spinach leaves or curly endive leaves
1 head chicory, broken into leaves
50 ml toasted and chopped hazelnuts and snipped fresh chives to garnish

DRESSING
1 medium onion, peeled and very finely chopped
1 clove garlic, crushed
15 ml white wine vinegar
salt and freshly ground black pepper
100 ml olive oil or canola oil
1 large Granny Smith apple, cored and finely chopped

Combine the dressing ingredients in a screw-top jar and shake well.
Arrange the watercress, lettuces, spinach and chicory in a large salad bowl. Top with the nuts and chives. Serve with the dressing.
375 kJ per serving

● High in fibre.

Suitable for: low gluten, low fat (reduce the quantity of oil to 50 ml), low cholesterol (reduce the quantity of oil to 50 ml).

Moroccan couscous salad

(Serves 6)

A substantial salad that's quick to prepare and keeps well.

500 g ripe tomatoes, skinned
3-4 spring onions, thinly sliced
15 ml canola oil
4 ml ground cumin
1 ml ground turmeric
pinch ground cinnamon
65 ml currants
45 ml finely chopped parsley
200 ml water
300 ml couscous
parsley, mint or coriander sprigs to garnish

Chop the tomatoes and leave to drain through a fine sieve. Sauté the spring onions in heated oil in a frying pan over moderate heat, stirring, for 1 minute. Stir in the cumin, turmeric, cinnamon, tomatoes, currants, chopped parsley and water.
Bring to the boil, then stir in the couscous and leave mixture to stand, covered, off the stove for 5 minutes, or until the couscous has absorbed the liquid. Leave to cool. Serve garnished with parsley, mint or coriander.
505 kJ per serving

● High in fibre.

Suitable for: low fat, low cholesterol.

Orange and olive salad with mustard dressing

(Serves 4-6)

An intriguing combination of flavours makes this salad a winner.

1 large onion, peeled and thinly sliced
3 large oranges, peeled and thickly sliced
500 ml watercress sprigs
18 pitted black olives
MUSTARD DRESSING
50 ml olive oil

2 ml mustard powder
1 ml castor sugar
45 ml white vinegar

Boil the onion uncovered, for 30 seconds. Drain, then rinse under cold water. Arrange the onion, orange slices, watercress and olives on a platter. Place the dressing in the centre. To make the dressing, place all the ingredients in a screw-top jar and shake well.
340 kJ per serving

● High in fibre.

Suitable for: low gluten.

Celery and red pepper salad with minted orange dressing

(Serves 2)

3 stalks celery, trimmed
1 medium red sweet pepper, cored and seeded
15 ml butter or canola oil
1 medium onion, peeled and finely chopped
30 ml pine kernels

DRESSING
5 ml grated orange peel
65 ml orange juice
15 ml canola oil
15 ml chopped fresh mint
2 ml sugar

Cut the celery and pepper into 5 cm long strips. Heat the butter or oil in a frying pan, add the onion and stir-fry until softened. Add the celery, red pepper and pine kernels and stir for 1 minute. Transfer to a large bowl. Add the dressing and toss well. Refrigerate for 30 minutes before serving.
To make the dressing, place all the ingredients in a screw-top jar and shake well.
495 kJ per serving

● High in fibre.

Suitable for: low gluten, low cholesterol (use oil).

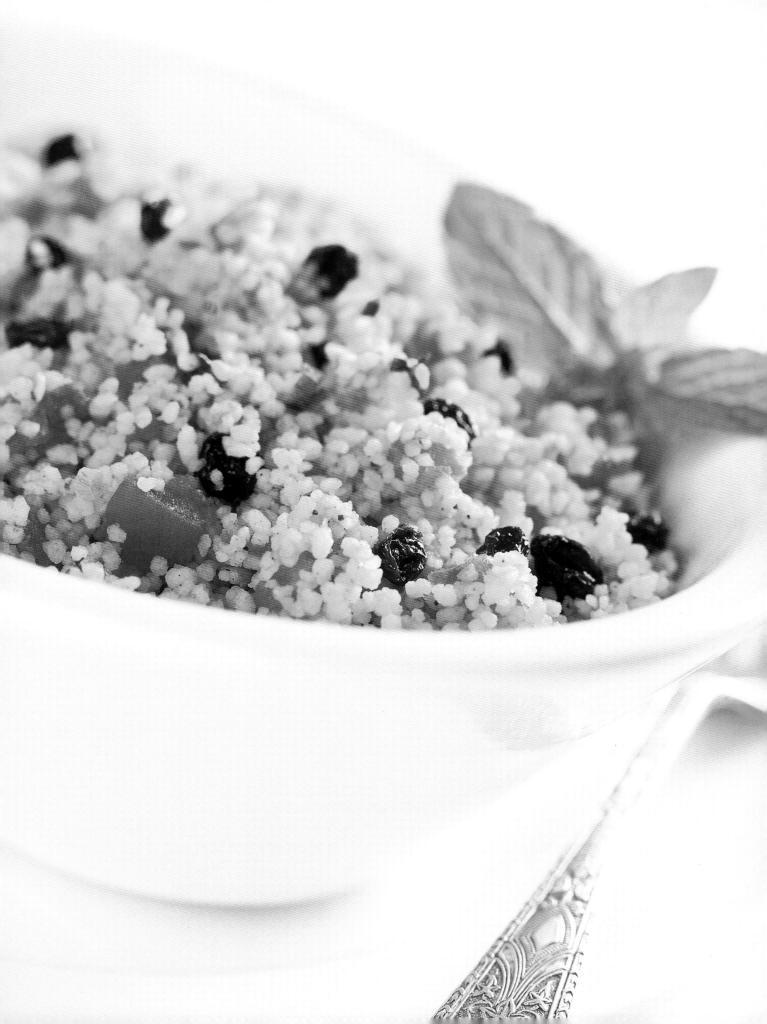

Cucumber ribbons with fresh tomato coulis

(Serves 4-6)

It's cool and delicious, and pretty as a picture – perfect for the buffet table.

2 English cucumbers, halved lengthways and seeds discarded
15 ml salt

COULIS
500 g large ripe tomatoes, skinned, seeded and chopped
3 spring onions, trimmed and thinly sliced
1 large clove garlic, crushed
5 ml seeded and puréed red sweet pepper (optional)
15 ml white wine vinegar
1 ml sugar
30 ml olive or canola oil
salt and freshly ground black pepper

Cut the cucumbers lengthways into thin strips, using a vegetable peeler, to make ribbons. Toss in a bowl with the salt and set aside for 10 minutes.
To make the coulis, combine the ingredients in a bowl, and season to taste with salt and pepper.
Drain the cucumbers in a colander, rinse well under cold water and pat dry with absorbent paper. Arrange on a serving platter and mound the coulis in the centre.
100 kJ per serving

Suitable for: low fat, low cholesterol.

Potato salad with yoghurt dressing

(Serves 4)

This lower-fat version makes a perennial favourite a guilt-free option.

750 g potatoes, cooked, cooled, skinned and diced
½ small cucumber, peeled and diced
2 hard-boiled egg whites, coarsely grated
50 g celery, trimmed and diced
25 g green or red sweet pepper, cored, seeded and diced
25 g spring onions, trimmed and chopped

DRESSING
100 ml low-fat natural yoghurt
15 ml tarragon or wine vinegar
5 ml salt
freshly ground black pepper to taste
5 ml mustard powder
5 ml chopped fresh mixed herbs

Toss the potatoes with the cucumber, egg whites, celery, green or red pepper and spring onions.
To make the dressing, combine the yoghurt with the vinegar, salt and pepper, mustard powder and herbs. Pour over the potatoes, then toss to combine and chill for 1 hour before serving.
460 kJ per serving

● High in fibre.

Suitable for: low fat, low cholesterol, low gluten, low sodium (omit the salt).

Vegetables

Mineral- and vitamin-rich vegetables and fruit are the first line of defence in the healthy diet. Use the freshest ingredients you can find (or even better, grow some yourself and harvest when you need them) to ensure optimum nutrient levels, not to mention the best taste around.

VEGETABLE SIDE DISHES
Forget about boring steamed, grilled or boiled vegetables served with meals – our tasty and unusual recipes will perk up any plate of food!

Roasted winter vegetables

(Serves 4)

250 g butternut, peeled and cut into chunks
1 large onion, peeled and quartered
250 g baby marrows, topped and tailed and cut
   into chunks
3 sweet potatoes, peeled and cut into chips
1 whole mealie, cut into chunks
2 cloves garlic, peeled
50 ml extra-virgin olive oil
5 ml mixed dried herbs
salt and coarsely ground black pepper

Preheat the oven to 200 °C.
Place all the vegetables in a roasting pan and drizzle
with olive oil. Sprinkle the herbs, salt and pepper over.
Bake for 45-60 minutes, or until crisp.
550 kJ per serving

Suitable for: low gluten, low sodium (omit salt).

Herbed green beans with garlic

(Serves 4)

Broad beans may be used instead of green beans.

500 g green beans, topped and tailed
5 ml olive oil
1 small onion, peeled and thinly sliced
1 clove garlic, crushed
15 ml chopped fresh thyme or oregano
salt and freshly ground black pepper to taste

Cook the beans in rapidly boiling water for 4-5 minutes,
or until crisp-tender. Drain.
In a heavy-based saucepan, heat the oil, add the onion
and garlic and sauté until the onion is softened but not
browned. Stir in the beans, thyme and salt and pepper
to taste. Heat through and serve.
220 kJ per serving

● High in fibre.

Suitable for: low gluten, low cholesterol, low fat.

Skewered vegetables

(Serves 6)

Vegetables threaded onto skewers and then braaied or
grilled make excellent accompaniments to meat, chicken or fish.

1 large brinjal, trimmed and cut into 1 cm cubes
6 medium tomatoes, quartered
250 g button mushrooms, trimmed
2 green sweet peppers, cored, seeded and cut into
   large pieces

BASTING MIXTURE
1 clove garlic, crushed
30 ml canola or olive oil
2 ml salt
freshly ground black pepper

Preheat the grill.
First make the basting mixture. Combine the garlic with
the oil, salt and a little pepper in a bowl.
Thread the vegetables onto 6 skewers, and brush well
with the oil mixture.
Grill the vegetables until tender, turning often and basting
2-3 times with the oil mixture. Serve at once.
290 kJ per serving

● High in fibre.
● Before making the kebabs, slice the brinjal thickly
and sprinkle with salt. Allow to draw for 20 minutes,
then fry lightly on both sides in oil. Cut into cubes.

VARIATIONS
● BRAAI THE KEBABS OVER HOT COALS.
● ADD OTHER VEGETABLES OF YOUR CHOICE, E.G. BABY
TOMATOES OR PARBOILED SMALL ONIONS.
● SERVE WITH GARLIC BUTTER, BUT NOTE THAT THIS
WILL ADD APPRECIABLY TO THE KILOJOULE AND FAT
COUNT OF THE DISH.

Suitable for: low cholesterol.

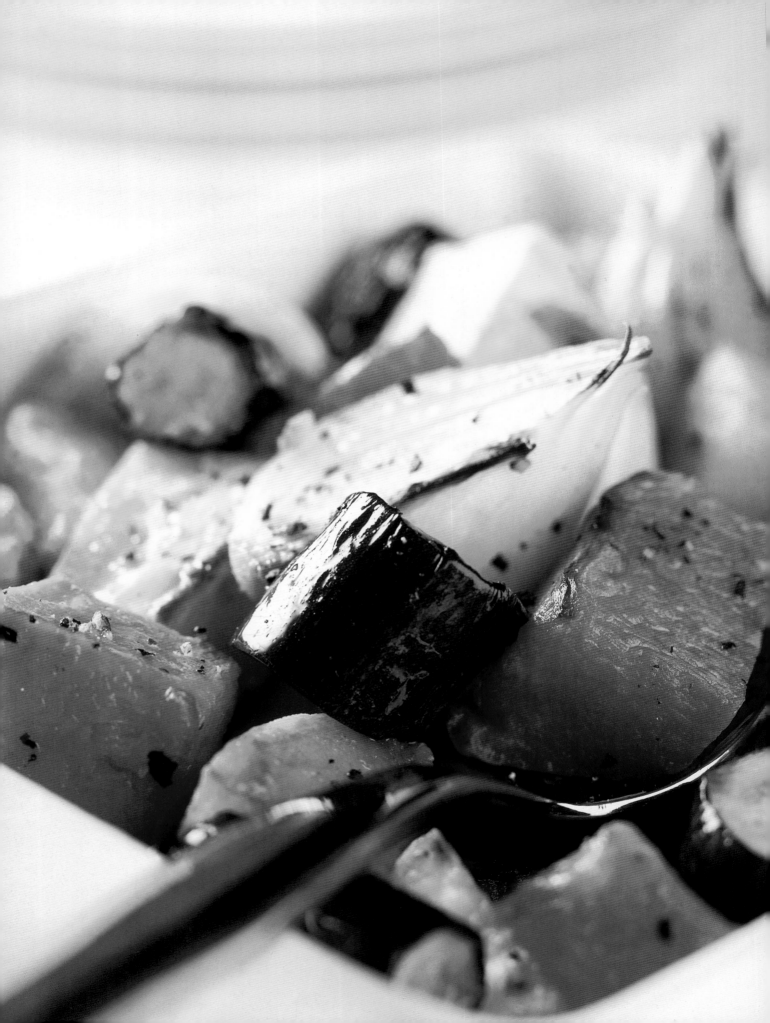

Low-gluten rösti

(Serves 4)

Boiling the potatoes in their jackets ensures that all the nutrients are retained.

600 g potatoes
knob of butter
15 ml extra-virgin olive oil
salt and pepper to taste

Boil the potatoes in their jackets for 10 minutes (do not overcook). Drain and set aside to cool. Peel the potatoes and grate them coarsely.
Heat the butter and oil in a 20 cm diameter nonstick frying pan. Spread the grated potatoes out evenly in the pan and pat down firmly. Reduce the heat, season with salt and pepper and cook for 10 minutes.
Invert a plate over the frying pan and turn the rösti out onto it, then slide the rösti back into the pan and cook on the other side. Divide the rösti into 4 portions and serve.
670 kJ per serving

Suitable for: low gluten, low cholesterol.

Potato gratin

(Serves 4)

Sage or oregano are also good herbs to use in this dish.

4 large potatoes, peeled and cut into 2 cm thick
   slices
4 medium onions, peeled and thinly sliced
2 cloves garlic, crushed
15 ml extra-virgin olive oil
15 ml chopped fresh thyme or 5 ml dried
2 ml salt
2 ml paprika
freshly ground black pepper to taste
125 ml low-fat milk

Preheat the oven to 200 °C.
Layer the potatoes in an ovenproof dish and sprinkle the onion and garlic over. Drizzle oil over, then sprinkle with herbs and seasoning. Pour over the milk and bake for 30-45 minutes, or until golden.
700 kJ per serving

● High in fibre.

Suitable for: low cholesterol, low fat.

Potato hedgehogs

(Serves 4-6)

This dish is known by many different names, but this one is perhaps the most descriptive.

6 medium baking potatoes
30 ml extra-virgin olive oil
5 ml salt

TOPPING 1
1 clove garlic, crushed
30 ml finely chopped onion

TOPPING 2
15 ml chopped parsley
5 ml chopped rosemary
5 ml chopped basil or oregano

TOPPING 3
5 ml paprika
2 ml cayenne pepper
2 ml ground cumin

Preheat the oven to 200 °C.
Scrub the potatoes well. Slice each potato thinly crossways, but do not cut all the way through. Place the potatoes in a baking pan. Fan the slices slightly, brush with oil and sprinkle with salt. Bake for 45-60 minutes, or until crisp and browned. Mix the ingredients for the topping of your choice and spoon it over the potatoes. Bake for another 10 minutes.
675 kJ per serving

● High in fibre.

Suitable for: low gluten, low cholesterol.

Baby marrows with mint pesto
(Serves 4)

The original pesto – basil and pine kernels instead of mint and walnuts – would also be a good choice here.

50 ml olive or canola oil
500 ml whole-kernel corn
2 ripe tomatoes, seeds discarded and flesh
  chopped
salt and freshly ground black pepper to taste
4 large baby marrows

PESTO
750 ml tightly packed fresh mint leaves
3 small cloves garlic, crushed
200 ml chopped walnuts
75 ml grated Parmesan cheese
salt to taste
150 ml extra-virgin olive oil or canola oil

First make the mint pesto. Purée the mint leaves, garlic, walnuts, Parmesan cheese and salt in a food processor or blender. With the motor running, add the oil in a steady stream, to make a smooth mixture. Transfer the pesto to a bowl, cover with plastic wrap and chill for 30 minutes.
Heat 50 ml oil in a large heavy-based frying pan and stir-fry the corn for 1 minute. Add the tomatoes and salt and pepper to taste and stir to combine. Transfer the mixture to a bowl.
Trim and halve the baby marrows lengthways. Scoop out and discard the seeds. Steam the shells for 3-5 minutes, or until barely tender, then drain on absorbent paper and allow to cool.
Spread about 7 ml pesto in each baby marrow shell and top with the corn and tomato mixture. Spoon more pesto mixture over, in 3 diagonal strips, each about 1 cm wide. Serve at room temperature.
250 kJ per serving

● High in fibre.

● This recipe may be prepared up to 3 hours in advance and stored, covered, at room temperature.

Suitable for: low gluten.

Oven-roasted potatoes with onions and rosemary
(Serves 4)

To impart a Mediterranean flavour, add a couple of pitted black olives and sliced red sweet pepper.

500 g large unpeeled potatoes, scrubbed
2 onions, peeled
3 cloves garlic, peeled
salt and coarsely ground black pepper to taste
125 ml rosemary sprigs
45 ml olive oil

Preheat the oven to 200 °C.
Cut the potatoes into eighths and quarter the onions. Spoon into a roasting pan and add the garlic, salt and pepper and rosemary. Drizzle with olive oil and roast for 30 minutes, or until crisp.
500 kJ per serving

● High in fibre.

Suitable for: low gluten, low sodium (omit salt), low cholesterol.

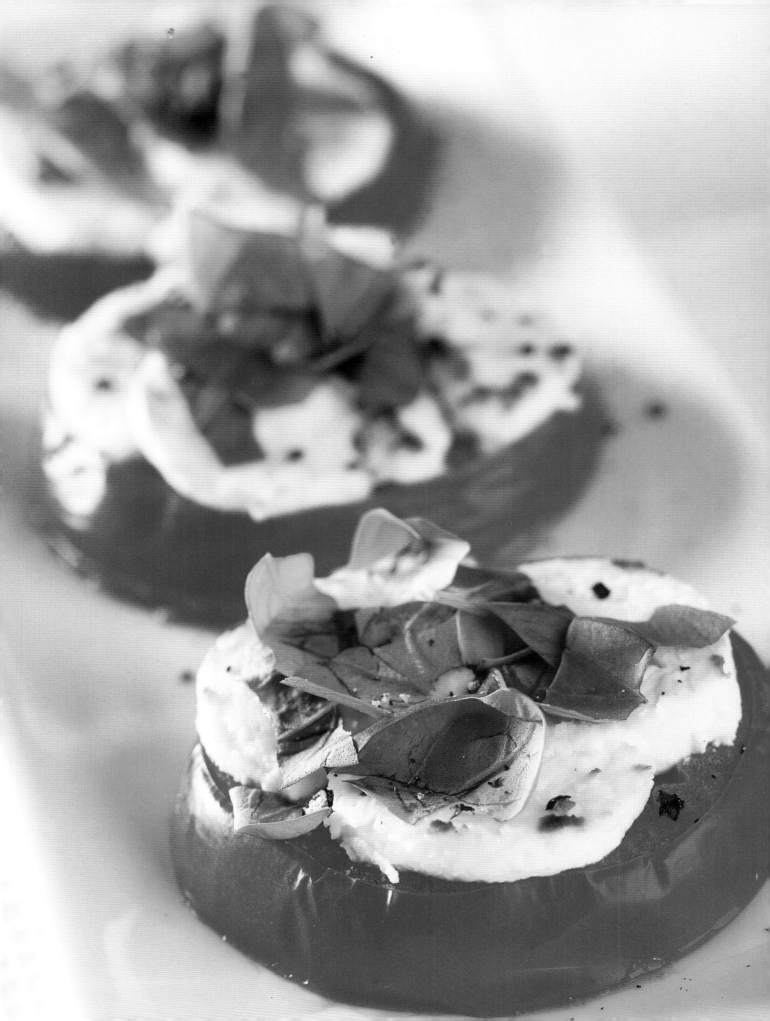

Grilled tomatoes with goat's milk cheese and basil

(Serves 4-6)

This is an excellent choice for serving with braaied or grilled lamb chops.

4 large ripe tomatoes
90 g chèvre (goat's milk cheese)
freshly ground black pepper to taste
45 ml chopped fresh basil

Preheat the grill.
Cut each tomato into 3-4 thick slices. Arrange in a single layer in a shallow baking dish. Slice the cheese thinly and arrange over the tomatoes. Sprinkle with pepper to taste, then basil, and grill for 2-3 minutes.
245 kJ per serving

To cook in the microwave: Arrange the tomato slices in a microwave-safe dish. Arrange the cheese on top, season and add the basil. Microwave on 100% power for 2 minutes, or until the cheese melts.

VARIATION: LOW-FAT MOZZARELLA OR TUSSERS MAY BE USED INSTEAD OF GOAT'S MILK CHEESE.

Suitable for: low fat, low cholesterol, low gluten.

Warm vegetable ribbons with chilli plum glaze

(Serves 4)

2 large baby marrows, topped and tailed
2 large carrots, peeled
2 large parsnips, peeled
15 ml sesame seeds, toasted

GLAZE
1 ml sesame or walnut oil
1 clove garlic, crushed
65 ml plum sauce
5 ml light soy sauce
5 ml chilli sauce
15 ml water

Trim or peel vegetables and cut into 8 cm lengths. Carefully cut thin 'ribbons' from each, using a vegetable peeler. Steam or microwave the vegetables until just tender and drain well.
Combine the oil, garlic, sauces and water for the glaze in a small saucepan. Stir over moderate heat for about 1 minute, or until heated through.
Toss the vegetable ribbons and glaze in a large bowl, sprinkle with the toasted sesame seeds and serve immediately.
750 kJ per serving

- Plum sauce is available from delis and oriental grocery stores.
- High in fibre.

To cook the glaze in the microwave: Place the glaze ingredients in a microwave-safe dish and microwave on 100% power for about 1 minute, or until heated through.

Suitable for: low cholesterol, low fat.

Warm carrot mousses with spinach sauce

(Serves 6)

A marvellous way to serve carrots — especially with chicken dishes.

45 ml butter, margarine or canola margarine
3 cloves garlic, crushed
7 medium carrots, peeled and sliced
375 ml chicken stock or low-salt chicken stock (recipe on page 149)
65 ml fresh coriander leaves
3 eggs, lightly beaten

SAUCE
6 large spinach leaves
250 ml white sauce or light white sauce (recipe on page 150)

Preheat the oven to 160 °C.
Heat the butter or margarine in a saucepan, add the garlic and carrots and stir until lightly browned. Add the chicken stock and bring to the boil, then reduce the heat

and simmer, covered, until tender. Strain the carrots, reserving 65 ml stock.

Purée the carrots, reserved stock and coriander until smooth. Cool the mixture slightly, then stir in the eggs.

Spoon the mixture into 6 x 125 ml greased moulds, place in a baking pan and add enough hot water to come halfway up the sides of the moulds. Bake for 40 minutes, or until just set.

Turn the mousses out onto serving plates and serve with spinach sauce.

To make the sauce, shred the spinach leaves, discarding the ribs, and wash well. Steam the spinach in the water clinging to the leaves until wilted, then drain well. Purée the spinach, and mix with the white sauce.

500 kJ per serving

VARIATIONS
- FRESH ASPARAGUS, STEAMED AND THEN PURÉED AND SEASONED, MAY BE USED INSTEAD OF THE SPINACH SAUCE.
- SERVE WITH FRESH TOMATO SAUCE (RECIPE ON PAGE 101 – CHICKEN AND SPINACH TERRINE).

Suitable for: low sodium (use low-salt chicken stock), low gluten.

Honeyed white onions
(Serves 4)

The caramelised onions look spectacular, but are really easy to make.

250 ml water
250 ml chicken stock or low-salt chicken stock (recipe on page 149)
700 g small white onions, peeled
30 ml canola oil
1 leek, trimmed and very finely chopped
1 clove garlic, crushed
5 ml lemon juice
dash cayenne pepper
pinch ground ginger
1 ml crushed mixed marjoram and tarragon leaves
15 ml honey

Preheat the oven to 180 °C.

Bring the water and stock to the boil in a heavy-based saucepan. Add the onions and cook, partially covered, for 15 minutes, or until almost tender. Drain.

Heat the oil in a nonstick frying pan. Add the leek and garlic and cook for 3 minutes, or until softened but not brown.

Arrange the onions in a lightly oiled, shallow baking dish. Sprinkle with lemon juice, cayenne pepper, ground ginger, herbs and the sautéed garlic and leek. Drizzle the honey over and bake for 20 minutes, turning the onions twice. Serve immediately.

630 kJ per serving

- High in fibre.

Suitable for: low cholesterol, low fat, low gluten, low sodium (use low-salt chicken stock).

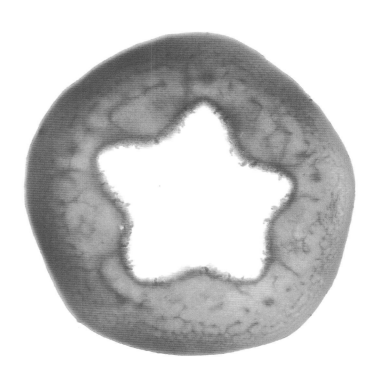

You don't have to be a vegetarian to enjoy a robust vegetable main meal. Put these recipes to the test – we're sure you'll love them.

Spicy vegetable tacos
(Serves 4)

For a totally different flavour, use steamed butternut or orange-fleshed pumpkin instead of sweet potatoes and grated nutmeg instead of chilli flakes and curry paste.

4 whole-wheat tortillas (recipe on page 136)

FILLING
300 g sweet potatoes, peeled and cubed
1 x 400 g can peeled tomatoes
1 x 400 g can chickpeas, drained
2 ml dried chilli flakes
30 ml mild curry paste
100 g spinach leaves
30 ml chopped fresh coriander
salt and pepper to taste
60 ml low-fat natural yoghurt

For the filling, cook the sweet potatoes in boiling water for 10-12 minutes, or until tender. Meanwhile, put the tomatoes, chickpeas, chilli flakes and curry paste in another saucepan and simmer for about 5 minutes. Preheat the grill.
Drain the sweet potatoes and add to the tomato mixture. Stir in the spinach and cook for 1 minute, or until just starting to wilt. Stir in the coriander, season to taste and keep warm.
Grill the tortillas for 20-30 seconds a side, spoon the filling onto one half, top with the yoghurt and fold over.
450 kJ per serving

● High in fibre.

Suitable for: low cholesterol, low fat, low gluten.

Bean burrito
(Serves 1)

Make a supply of refried beans and store, ready to be used for burritos or simply on their own. Refried beans provide plenty of fibre.

REFRIED BEANS
(Makes about 1 kg)

375 ml uncooked kidney beans
65 ml chopped onion
2 cloves garlic, crushed
15 ml canola oil
5 ml ground cumin

Soak the beans overnight in water to cover. The next day, boil the beans in 1,5 litres of water until tender, 2-3 hours. Drain, reserving some of the liquid.
Sauté the onion and garlic in the heated oil. Mash half the beans and add to the onions and garlic. Fry the mixture, then add some whole beans and the cumin, as well as some of the cooking liquid to keep the bean mixture soft.
To make 1 burrito, heat 125 ml refried beans and add 10-15 ml chopped chillies (optional). Spoon the mixture onto 1 whole-wheat tortilla (recipe on page 136), then heap 30 ml chopped peeled tomato, 2 shredded lettuce leaves and 30 ml low-fat natural yoghurt on top. Fold the tortilla over and serve.
950 kJ per serving

● If you're not on a sodium-restricted diet, add salt to the bean mixture, or use canned beans (to save time).

Suitable for: low sodium, low cholesterol.

Vegetable paella
(Serves 4)

Other vegetables could also be used – brinjals, baby marrows and mushrooms, for example.

50 ml extra-virgin olive oil
250 g uncooked rice
3 large onions, peeled and finely chopped

1 large clove garlic, crushed with 5 ml salt
3 large tomatoes, skinned and coarsely chopped
1 ml saffron or turmeric soaked in 600 ml hot water or stock (omit salt)
120 g cucumber, peeled and diced
3 stalks celery, trimmed and finely chopped
1 large green sweet pepper, cored, seeded and thinly sliced
15 ml finely chopped fresh parsley
15 ml finely chopped fresh thyme
5 ml grated lemon peel
5 ml salt
2 ml pepper
6 stoned black olives, thin red sweet pepper strips and fresh bean sprouts to garnish

Heat the oil in a heavy-based frying pan and stir-fry the rice until it turns pale yellow. Add the onions and garlic and sauté for 3 minutes. Add the tomatoes and the saffron and water mixture, then reduce the heat and simmer, covered, for 15 minutes.

Stir in the cucumber and celery and simmer for 5 minutes. Add the green pepper and simmer until the rice is just tender and all the liquid has been absorbed, about 5 minutes. Add more hot water if the mixture is too dry. Remove from the stove and stir in the parsley, thyme and lemon peel, adding more salt and pepper if necessary. Turn the mixture into a serving dish and garnish with the olives and red pepper strips. Serve with fresh sprouts sprinkled on top.
620 kJ per serving
● This dish is rich in fibre.

VARIATIONS
● ADD SLIVERED CHICKEN BREAST FILLETS WITH THE ONION AND GARLIC.
● ADD WHITE FISH STRIPS WITH THE ONION AND GARLIC.

Suitable for: low fat, low gluten.

Low-cholesterol vegetable frittata
(Serves 2)

The recipe may easily be doubled to serve four; use two frying pans.

10 ml canola oil
1 clove garlic, crushed
250 ml leftover cooked vegetables such as broccoli, beans, brinjals, corn kernels
7 ml mixed dried herbs
freshly ground black pepper to taste
175 ml egg substitute (recipe on page 150)
2 egg whites
30 ml grated Parmesan cheese or low-fat yellow cheese

Heat the oil in a frying pan and sauté the garlic until softened. Add the vegetables and herbs and cook briefly.
Beat the egg substitute and egg whites together, stir in the cheese and pour over vegetable mixture. Cook until golden underneath.
Turn over with a spatula and cook on the other side until golden, or place briefly under the grill to cook the top.
974 kJ per serving

● For a low-sodium frittata, use unsalted vegetables and omit the cheese.

Suitable for: low cholesterol.

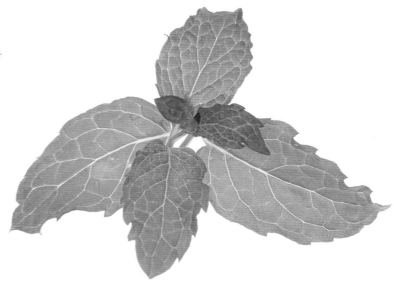

Ricotta roulade with fresh tomato sauce

(Serves 8)

An excellent lunch dish, served with salads of your choice.

250 g low-fat ricotta cheese
250 g low-fat creamed cottage cheese
65 ml grated Parmesan cheese
20 ml chopped fresh basil
1 clove garlic, crushed
1 bacon rasher, finely chopped
15 ml gelatine powder
30 ml water
18 stuffed olives
20 spinach leaves
fresh tomato sauce (Spaghetti with fresh tomato sauce, page 127)

Beat the ricotta and cottage cheese together until smooth. Stir in the Parmesan cheese, basil and garlic. Fry the bacon until crisp, then drain on absorbent paper.
Sprinkle the gelatine over the water in a container, and stand it in a small pan of simmering water until dissolved, stirring constantly. Cool to room temperature but do not allow to set.
Add the bacon, gelatine mixture and olives to the cheeses and mix well.
Steam or microwave the spinach until wilted, then rinse under cold water and pat dry. Lay the spinach leaves in a single layer, slightly overlapping, on a 15 x 30 cm sheet of plastic wrap. Spoon the cheese mixture on the long side of spinach, leaving a 5 cm border. Fold in the ends of the spinach and roll up like a Swiss roll, using the plastic to lift and guide the roll. Wrap securely in foil. Refrigerate for a few hours, preferably overnight. Serve, sliced, with fresh tomato sauce.
880 kJ per serving

● The olives in the roulade and the sauce may be omitted.

To sponge the gelatine in the microwave: Microwave on 100% power for 20 seconds.

Suitable for: low fat, low cholesterol.

Upside-down tomato and caramelised onion tart

(Serves 4)

This tart is a savoury version of a tarte tatin (inverted apple tart), and absolutely delicious.

PASTRY
85 g butter
175 g self-raising flour
50 g grated Parmesan cheese
fresh thyme leaves
salt
1 large egg yolk
30 ml cold water

CARAMELISED ONIONS
15 ml butter
15 ml olive oil
1 large onion, cut into rounds
5 ml sugar

GARLIC TOMATOES
15 ml extra-virgin olive oil
5 ml sugar
1 fat clove garlic, peeled and thinly sliced
5 large Roma tomatoes, halved lengthways
fresh thyme sprigs
300 g cherry tomatoes

First prepare the onions. Heat the butter and oil in a frying pan until melted. Fry the onion over moderate heat for about 10 minutes, or until golden, stirring often. Stir in the sugar and cook for a further 1-2 minutes. Tip the onions and their juices into a bowl and set aside.
Preheat the oven to 200 °C.
To make the pastry, rub the butter into the flour to make a fine crumbly mixture. Stir in the cheese, thyme and a little salt, then add the egg yolk and cold water. Mix to make a dough. Wrap in cling film.
To make the tomatoes, heat the oil in a 20 cm diameter tarte tatin pan, or a shallow metal pie dish, on top of the stove. Stir in the sugar and garlic, then add the tomatoes, cut side down, and interleave with thyme sprigs. Cook for 1 minute. Scatter whole cherry tomatoes over the base and remove from the stove.

Spread the onions on top, season and set aside.
Roll out the pastry until slightly larger than the top of the pan. Lay over the onions and tuck any excess down the sides of the pan.

Place on a baking sheet and bake for 25 minutes, or until the pastry is golden. Cool for 5 minutes, then place a heated plate, upside down, over the pan. Invert, shaking to loosen the tart onto the plate. Sprinkle extra thyme over and season with black pepper. Serve hot.

1 625 kJ per serving

Ratatouille

(Serves 4-6)

Ratatouille may also be cooked on top of the stove, and is delicious served cold.

1 medium brinjal, thickly sliced
course salt
75 ml olive or canola oil
3 baby marrows, thinly sliced
3 large, firm tomatoes, thinly sliced
1 large onion, peeled and thickly sliced
1 green or yellow sweet
**   pepper, cored,**
**   seeded and sliced**

200 g mushrooms, wiped and thinly sliced
3 cloves garlic, crushed
2 ml each dried oregano and thyme
5 ml salt
2 ml freshly ground black pepper
grated Parmesan cheese (optional)

Sprinkle the brinjal with coarse salt and leave to draw for 30 minutes. Rinse and pat dry.
Preheat the oven to 180 °C.
Heat the oil in a large frying pan and sauté the brinjal and baby marrow slices until lightly browned. Place in a greased casserole dish.
Layer the tomatoes, onion, sweet pepper and mushrooms over the brinjals and baby marrows, sprinkling each layer with garlic, thyme and oregano. Sprinkle the salt and pepper over the top layer.
Bake, uncovered, for 1 hour. Serve hot, with Parmesan cheese, if desired.

500 kJ per serving

● High in fibre.

Suitable for: low cholesterol, low gluten.

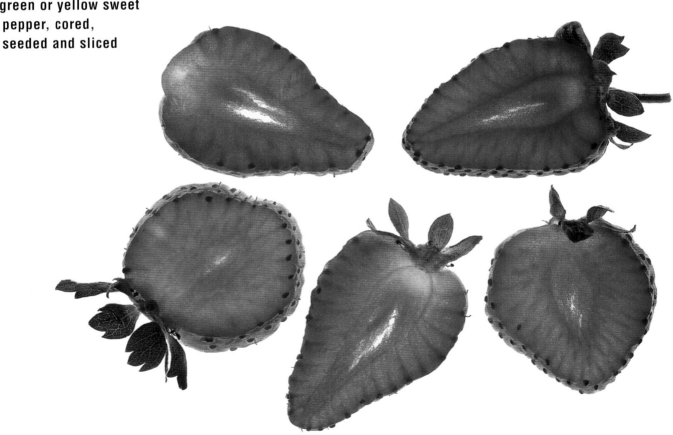

Spinach and mushroom lasagne

(Serves 6)

a pasta dish with a rich, robust flavour.

250 g fresh or dried lasagne sheets
350 g spinach, shredded
225 g baby button mushrooms
45 ml water
5 ml salt
350 g cottage cheese
10 ml grated Parmesan cheese

SAUCE
30 ml cornflour or arrowroot
150 ml milk
1 x 400 g can tomatoes
2 ml lemon juice
2 ml grated nutmeg
5 ml salt

Preheat the oven to 220 °C.

Cook the lasagne sheets according to package instructions. Drain thoroughly.

Place the spinach, mushrooms, water and salt in a saucepan. Bring to the boil, stirring, then reduce the heat and simmer, uncovered, for 25-30 minutes, or until most of the liquid has evaporated.

To make the tomato sauce, tip the cornflour into a clean saucepan and blend until smooth with a little milk. Stir in the remaining milk and cook, stirring, until the mixture thickens. Simmer for 1 minute. Stir in the chopped tomatoes and the lemon juice. Bring to the boil, stirring often, then mix in the nutmeg and salt.

Layer the lasagne sheets, spinach mixture, tomato sauce and cottage cheese alternately into a lightly oiled 23 cm diameter, 6 cm deep, dish. Start and end with lasagne sheets.

Sprinkle with Parmesan cheese and bake for 25 minutes.

920 kJ per serving

- Arrowroot doesn't leave the slight aftertaste in a sauce that cornflour does.
- This dish is rich in fibre.

Suitable for: low gluten, low fat, low cholesterol.

Vegetable and chickpea curry

(Serves 6)

The combination of spices makes this curry aromatic rather than strong, and definitely moreish.

15 ml canola oil
5 ml black mustard seeds
5 ml turmeric
15 ml garam masala
10 ml cumin
seeds from 6 green cardamom pods
4 cloves
1 ml cayenne pepper
1 clove garlic, crushed
175 g onions, peeled and thinly sliced
350 g leeks, shredded
250 g carrots, peeled and thinly sliced
450 g potatoes or celeriac, peeled and cubed
250 g brinjals, cubed
250 g parsnips, peeled and cubed
600 ml boiling water
60 ml tomato purée
10 ml salt
1 x 425 g can chickpeas

Heat the oil until sizzling in a large saucepan. Add the spices and fry gently for 5 minutes, then leave the saucepan over low heat for about 5 minutes. Stir and add the garlic.

Add the vegetables to the saucepan and mix them in well. Mix the water with the tomato purée and salt. Pour over the vegetables and bring to the boil, stirring constantly.

Reduce the heat and simmer the curry, covered, for 45 minutes. Stir in the chickpeas and the canning liquid and simmer, covered, for a further 20 minutes. Serve with noodles or rice.

920 kJ per serving

- High in fibre.

Suitable for: low cholesterol, low fat, low gluten.

Poultry

The emphasis in this chapter is on turkey and chicken; both are versatile, leaner than duck and goose, and the excess fat is easy to remove – which are all useful in a healthy diet.

TURKEY

Turkey meat is a great protein source if you're watching your weight or have to cut down on fats in your diet, because it is fairly lean and lends itself to all kinds of interesting and tasty dishes. If you serve roast turkey as your holiday meat, there's always plenty left over, and you can use that meat for any of the recipes – turkey or chicken – given in this chapter.

Turkey salad with avocado dressing
(Serves 4)

A great recipe for using up leftovers. The avocado used is small, and won't add appre[c] fat content per serving.

250 g cooked turkey meat, chopped
**½ ripe papino or small sweet melon, pe[]
seeded and cubed**
**8 asparagus spears or 100 g young gree[]
beans, steamed and chopped**
500 g cooked new potatoes
2 celery stalks, trimmed and sliced
250 g cherry tomatoes
**1 red oak-leaf lettuce, separated i
nto leaves**

AVOCADO DRESSING
½ small avocado, peeled and stoned
1 garlic clove, crushed (optional)
10 ml balsamic vinegar
**30 ml crème fraîche, low-fat natural yoghurt or
low-fat cottage cheese**
salt and freshly ground black pepper to taste

Combine the turkey with the papino or melon, asparagus or beans, potatoes, celery and tomatoes and serve on a bed of lettuce. Drizzle the dressing over just before serving.

To make the dressing, blend all the ingredients together until smooth, seasoning to taste.

950 kJ per serving

● High in fibre.

VARIATION: LEFTOVER CHICKEN MAY BE USED INSTEAD OF TURKEY.

Suitable for: low gluten, low cholesterol (use low-fat natural yoghurt).

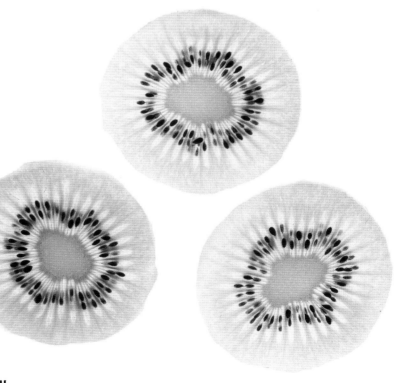

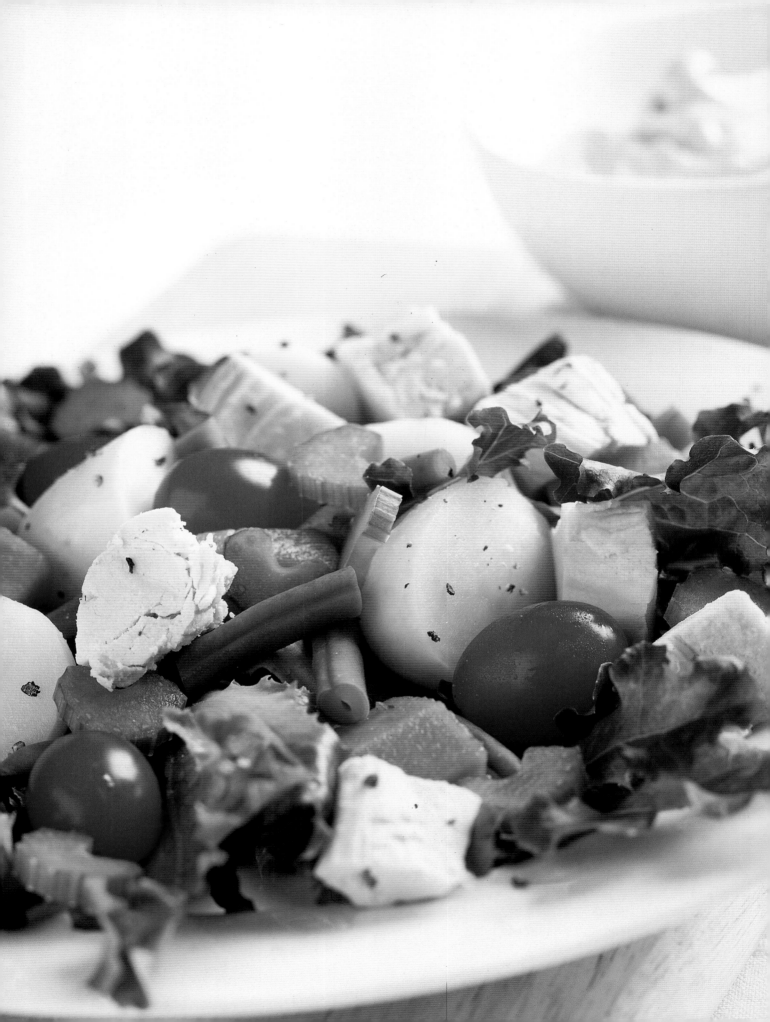

Turkey and mushroom pilaf
(Serves 4)

Use other vegetables, if you prefer; brinjals, sweet red peppers and baby marrows are a good combination.

5 ml extra-virgin olive oil
1 medium onion, peeled and finely chopped
1 green sweet pepper, cored, seeded and finely chopped
200 g uncooked arborio rice
500 ml chicken stock or low-salt chicken stock (recipe on page 149)
400 g leftover cooked turkey, coarsely chopped
100 g mushrooms, wiped and thinly sliced
2 ripe tomatoes, thinly sliced
salt and freshly ground black pepper to taste
chopped parsley or basil to garnish

Heat the oil in a large frying pan and sauté the onion and green pepper until tender. Add the rice and sauté for 2 minutes, then stir in the chicken stock, cover and simmer for 10 minutes.
Stir in the turkey, mushrooms and tomatoes, season and simmer for another 10 minutes. Serve at once, garnished with parsley or basil.
1 680 kJ per serving

VARIATION: USE COOKED CHICKEN INSTEAD OF TURKEY.

Suitable for: low gluten, low fat, low sodium (use low-salt chicken stock), low cholesterol.

Apricot and turkey kebabs with mustard basting sauce
(Serves 4)

Leftover cooked turkey may also be used.

125 g dried apricots
hot water
500 g boned turkey breast

BASTING SAUCE
15 ml Dijon mustard
30 ml lemon juice
7 ml extra-virgin olive oil

Soak the apricots in hot water to cover for 30 minutes. Drain thoroughly. Cube the turkey and thread onto 4 skewers, each 20 cm long, alternately with the apricots.
To make the basting sauce, beat together the mustard, lemon juice and oil.
Line a grilling pan with foil. Place the kebabs in the pan and brush with the basting sauce. Grill for a total of 15 minutes, turning the kebabs 4 times and brushing often with the remaining basting sauce. Serve with Green salad with apple dressing (recipe on page 77).
650 kJ per serving

● High in fibre.

VARIATIONS
● BRAAI THE KEBABS OVER THE COALS INSTEAD OF GRILLING.
● USE CUBED CHICKEN BREAST INSTEAD OF TURKEY.
● USE CUBED PORK FILLET INSTEAD OF TURKEY.

Turkey and pineapple kebabs: Omit the apricots. Thread the turkey onto 4 skewers alternately with ½ fresh pineapple, peeled and cubed, and 75 g button mushrooms, stalks removed. Prepare a basting sauce from 30 ml apple juice beaten with 15 ml clear honey, 15 ml Worcestershire sauce, 15 ml white vinegar, 10 ml oil and 5 ml salt. Proceed as described in the recipe.

Suitable for: low gluten, low fat, low cholesterol.

Remove the skin and the visible fat from chicken before cooking, and it becomes a good lower-fat choice. And if you use chicken breast fillets, you're guaranteed lean meat, which is why mainly breast fillets are used in these recipes.

Chicken fricassée

(Serves 4)

A quick and easy dish, prepared on top of the stove.

25 ml butter, margarine or canola oil
125 g mushrooms, wiped and thinly sliced
65 ml flour, cornflour or arrowroot
300 ml low-fat milk
250 g cooked chicken, cubed
125 g frozen peas
5 ml salt
2 ml pepper

Melt the butter or margarine, or heat the oil, in a large frying pan, add the mushrooms and sauté until tender. Remove the pan from the stove, stir in the flour and gradually blend in the milk.

Return the frying pan to the stove, bring the milk mixture to the boil and simmer, stirring all the time, until the sauce thickens.

Stir in the chicken cubes and the peas and simmer, stirring occasionally, until heated through, 5-10 minutes.

Season, then transfer the fricassée to a heated serving dish. Serve with mashed potatoes and steamed carrots and broccoli.

950 kJ per serving

● High in fibre.

Suitable for: low gluten (use cornflour or arrowroot), low cholesterol (use oil).

Chilled chicken breasts with lemon-dill sauce

(Serves 6)

A deliciously light sauce adds piquancy to this ideal summer dish.

6 chicken breast fillets
dill sprigs to garnish

SAUCE
50 ml semisweet white wine or unsweetened white grape juice
finely grated peel of 2 lemons
100 ml chicken stock or low-salt chicken stock (recipe on page 149)
125 ml chopped fresh dill
50 ml low-fat natural yoghurt

Start with the sauce. Heat the wine or grape juice to just below boiling point, add the lemon peel, cover and infuse overnight.

Next day, heat a nonstick frying pan and pack the chicken breasts in it in a single layer. Cook on one side only for 5-8 minutes. Remove from the pan and keep hot.

Place the lemon-flavoured wine and the stock in the pan and stir to mix. Add the dill and cook, uncovered, to reduce the sauce by about half. Stir in the yoghurt.

Sliver the chicken breasts and place in a serving dish. Pour the sauce over and chill. Garnish with dill sprigs and serve with a salad.

720 kJ per serving

Suitable for: low sodium (use low-salt chicken stock), low cholesterol, low fat, low gluten.

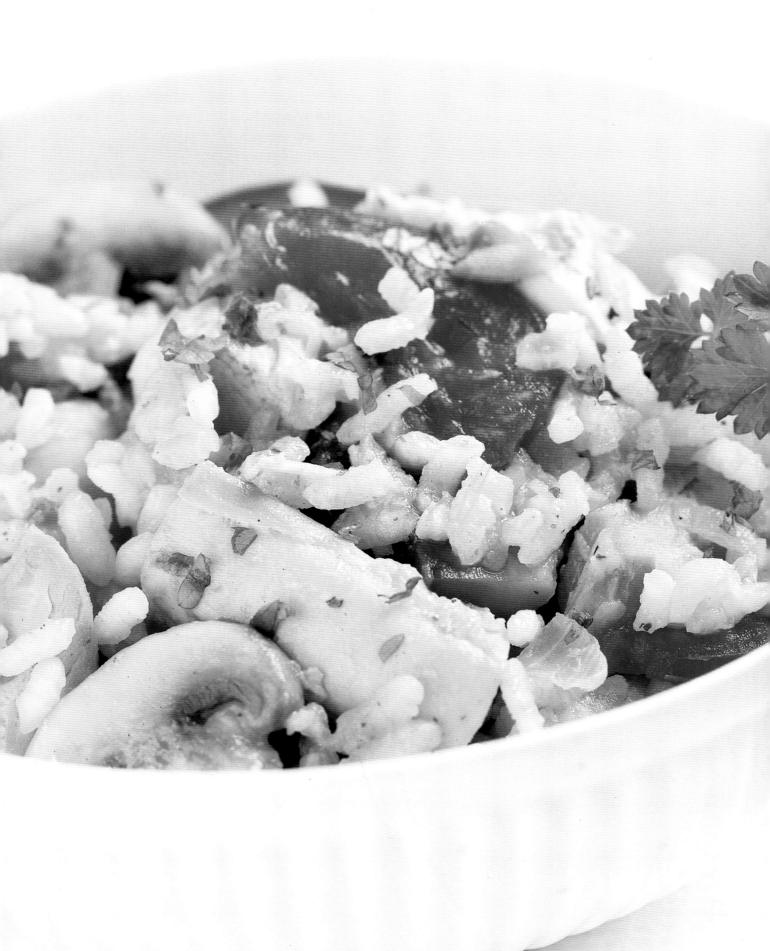

Peach chicken schnitzel

(Serves 4-5)

Lemon adds piquancy to chicken and for this reason the two are often combined; peaches, however, add a subtler nuance to the flavour of the chicken.

500 g chicken breast fillets
20-30 ml unsweetened peach juice
50 ml flour
2 ml salt
2 ml thyme
2 ml celery salt (optional)
1 egg
5 ml water
125 ml fine dried breadcrumbs

Preheat the oven to 200 °C.
Cut the chicken breasts horizontally into 5 mm thick slices. Place the breasts between 2 pieces of waxed paper and flatten them, using a meat mallet. Sprinkle with peach juice and let stand for 10 minutes.
Combine the flour, salt, thyme and celery salt (if using) in a shallow dish and mix well. In another shallow dish, lightly beat the egg with the water.
Dip the chicken pieces into the flour mixture, then into the egg mixture, then into breadcrumbs. Place on a lightly greased baking sheet and bake for 10-15 minutes, carefully turning once. Serve with new potatoes and steamed butternut.
1 150 kJ per serving

To cook in the microwave: Microwave the crumbed chicken schnitzels, uncovered, on 100% power for 4 minutes.

Suitable for: low fat, low cholesterol.

Chicken and asparagus bake

(Serves 4)

Fresh asparagus and chicken are a marriage made in heaven, but if fresh asparagus is unavailable, canned salad cuts will do.

5 ml canola or extra-virgin olive oil
1 small onion, peeled and very finely chopped
4 chicken breast fillets, cut into strips
400 g fresh young asparagus spears, steamed and cut into pieces
pinch cayenne pepper
salt and freshly ground black pepper to taste
½ portion mozzarella cheese sauce (recipe on page 149)

TOPPING
250 ml fresh whole-wheat breadcrumbs
50 ml shredded mozzarella cheese
pinch cayenne pepper
20 ml canola margarine, for dotting

Heat the oil in a frying pan and sauté the onion until softened but not browned. Add the chicken strips and stir-fry until cooked. Remove from the frying pan with a slotted spoon and transfer to a lightly oiled ovenproof dish. Add the asparagus cuts and season with cayenne pepper, salt and black pepper. Pour the cheese sauce over.
To make the topping, mix the breadcrumbs, mozzarella cheese and a little cayenne pepper together and sprinkle over the top. Dot with margarine and bake for 30 minutes, at 180º C, or until heated through and the topping is crisp. Serve immediately.
1 450 kJ per serving

Rosemary-baked chicken

(Serves 4-6)

1,5 kg chicken pieces
500 ml low-fat natural yoghurt
75 ml dried white breadcrumbs
75 ml grated Parmesan cheese
65 ml chopped fresh rosemary, or 45 ml dried
5 ml salt
5 ml freshly ground black pepper
2 ml paprika
1 egg, beaten
45 ml canola oil

Preheat the oven to 180 °C.

Place the chicken pieces in a large bowl and pour the yoghurt over. Refrigerate, covered, for 1 hour.

Combine the breadcrumbs, cheese, rosemary, salt, pepper and paprika in a dish.

Remove the chicken pieces from the yoghurt, dip them in beaten egg, then coat in the breadcrumb mixture. Place, skin side up, in an oiled baking dish and drizzle with oil. Bake for 50 minutes, or until crisp and brown, turning once. Drain on absorbent paper. Serve hot or cold, with noodles and steamed vegetables, or a salad.
1 200 kJ per serving

VARIATION: USE DRIED TARRAGON INSTEAD OF ROSEMARY.

Suitable for: low cholesterol (remove chicken skin before preparation).

Chicken, apple and red sweet pepper stir-fry
(Serves 4)

The combination of flavours in this stir-fry is absolute bliss – sweet and aromatic.

30 ml canola or extra-virgin olive oil
2 medium leeks, trimmed and sliced
4 chicken breast fillets, cut into thick strips
1 large or 2 smaller Starking or other crisp red apple(s), cored and sliced lengthways
1 red sweet pepper, cored, seeded and cut into strips
60 ml unsweetened granadilla or apricot juice
10 ml ground cinnamon
salt and freshly ground black pepper to taste
cooked noodles of your choice, to serve

Heat the oil in a large frying pan and sauté the leeks until softened but not browned. Pack the chicken strips in the pan, interspersing them with apple slices and sweet red pepper strips. Cook, undisturbed, for 1 minute, then stir-fry over moderate heat until the chicken is cooked and the apples and peppers are tender. Reduce the heat, add the granadilla or apricot juice and cook, partially covered, until most of the liquid has evaporated.

Remove the lid, season with the cinnamon and salt and pepper to taste, and stir-fry for a further 1-2 minutes. Serve immediately, on a bed of cooked noodles.
600 kJ per serving

VARIATION: USE PORK FILLET STRIPS INSTEAD OF CHICKEN.

Suitable for: low cholesterol, low fat, low gluten.

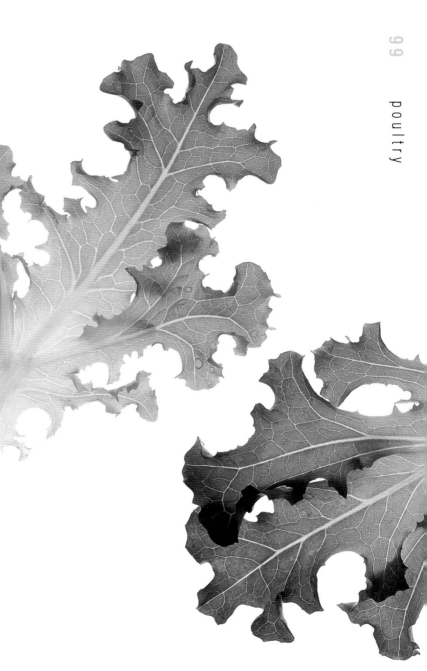

Chicken curry

(Serves 6)

Mild chicken curry is a perennial favourite, which can be adapted for lower-fat cooking by using chicken breast fillets instead of chicken pieces.

25 ml canola oil
1,5 kg chicken pieces
2 medium onions, peeled and finely chopped
500 ml chicken stock, or low-salt chicken stock
**   (recipe on page 149)**
30 ml curry powder
10 ml turmeric
10 ml ground coriander
125 ml seedless raisins
125 ml desiccated coconut
pinch sugar
pinch ground cinnamon
125 ml low-fat natural yoghurt or low-fat butter-
**   milk**
15 ml cornflour
15 ml brandy (optional)

Preheat the oven to 160 °C.
Heat the oil in a large saucepan and brown the chicken pieces and onions until golden brown.
Combine the stock, curry powder, turmeric, coriander, raisins, coconut, sugar and cinnamon in a bowl.
Transfer the chicken, onions and pan juices to a large casserole dish, then pour the curry mixture over.
Bake, covered, until tender, about 1 hour.
Mix together the yoghurt or buttermilk, cornflour and brandy in a small saucepan and simmer over medium heat, stirring constantly, until thickened.
Pour the sauce over the chicken and serve with boiled white or brown rice.
1 250 kJ per serving

- For low-cholesterol diets, skin the chicken pieces before frying, or use chicken breast fillets instead of chicken pieces.

Suitable for: low sodium (use low-salt chicken stock).

Tandoori chicken

(Serves 4)

This Indian dish was originally cooked in a tandoor (outdoor clay oven), but it's just as tasty grilled or braaied.

2 x 1 kg chickens
10 ml salt
50 ml canola or olive oil
1 ml turmeric or crumbled saffron threads

MARINADE
30 ml fresh lemon juice
10 ml ground coriander
5 ml ground cumin
250 ml low-fat natural yoghurt
1 onion, peeled and sliced
3 cloves garlic, crushed
15 ml peeled and chopped fresh ginger
5 ml ground cinnamon
2 ml turmeric or crumbled saffron threads
5 ml dried red chilli flakes or 2 ml chilli sauce

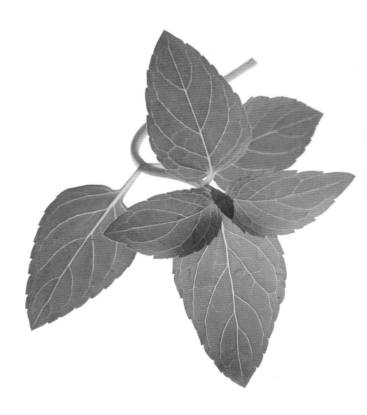

Halve the chickens and make incisions in the flesh with a sharp knife. Rub salt into the chickens and place them in a large, flat dish.

To make the marinade, mix all the ingredients. Spoon over the chickens and marinate for at least 5 hours, but preferably overnight.

Remove the chickens from the marinade and brush with the oil mixed with the turmeric or saffron. Grill for 5 minutes on each side to seal in juices, then reduce the heat (or lower the pan) and grill until cooked, about 30 minutes. Serve with yellow rice or couscous and sambals.

1 250 kJ per serving

- Tandoori chicken may also be braaied over the coals.
- To cut down on the fat content, remove the chicken skin before marinating, reduce the quantity of oil to 25 ml and serve the chicken with boiled white or brown rice.
- The marinade may be thickened with 10 ml cornflour and served as a sauce with the chicken.

Chicken and spinach terrine

(Serves 4-6)

Layers of spinach and chicken in a spinach casing are served with a smooth, flavourful tomato sauce.

1 bunch young spinach leaves

CHICKEN FILLING
5 ml canola or extra-virgin olive oil
1 medium onion, peeled and finely chopped
2 bacon rashers, chopped
10 ml curry powder
4 chicken breast fillets, chopped
65 ml crème fraîche, low-fat natural yoghurt or
  light white sauce (recipe on page 150)
2 eggs

SPINACH FILLING
15 ml butter
1 clove garlic, crushed
1 bunch spinach, chopped
200 ml cooked rice

30 ml crème fraîche, low-fat natural yoghurt or
  light white sauce (recipe on page 150)
1 egg
1 ml grated nutmeg

TOMATO SAUCE
3 ripe tomatoes, skinned and chopped
1 medium onion, peeled and chopped
15 ml balsamic vinegar
2 ml sugar

Preheat the oven to 180 °C.

First make the chicken filling. Heat the oil in a frying pan, add the onion, bacon and curry powder and stir constantly over moderate heat until the onion is soft. Blend the onion mixture, chicken, crème fraîche and eggs until smooth.

SPINACH FILLING: Melt the butter in a saucepan, add the garlic and spinach and stir over low heat until the spinach is soft. Drain the spinach and press out as much moisture as possible. Combine with the rice, crème fraîche, egg and nutmeg in a bowl. Mix well.

Steam or microwave the spinach for lining the pan until tender; drain well. Line the base and sides of an oiled 12 x 23 cm ovenproof loaf pan (or spray it with nonstick spray) with spinach, reserving a few leaves for the top. Spread half the chicken mixture into the dish, top with the spinach filling and spread the remaining chicken filling on top. Cover with the reserved spinach leaves, then cover with foil.

Place the pan in a baking dish holding enough hot water to come halfway up the sides of the loaf pan. Bake for 1 hour, or until set. Remove the pan from the water and allow to stand for 5 minutes. Remove the foil and invert the terrine onto a serving dish. Serve warm or cold with tomato sauce.

TOMATO SAUCE: Combine all the ingredients in a saucepan and bring to the boil. Reduce the heat and simmer, covered, for 10 minutes. Purée until smooth, then strain. Reheat and serve with the terrine.

950 kJ per serving

Suitable for: low gluten, low fat (use yoghurt or light white sauce, recipe on page 150).

Chicken and nectarine salad

(Serves 4)

Celebrate summer with this luscious chicken, fruit and vegetable salad.

4 chicken breast fillets
150 ml unsweetened peach juice
100 ml chicken stock or low-salt chicken stock
  (recipe on page 149)
1-2 baby gem or cos lettuce, separated into leaves
¼ English cucumber, thinly sliced
4 ripe nectarines
16 baby mealies
10 ml cornflour or arrowroot
salt and freshly ground black pepper to taste
1 round herbed feta cheese, crumbled
parsley sprigs to garnish

Place the chicken breasts in a saucepan just large enough to take them comfortably. Mix the peach juice and the stock, pour it over the chicken and bring to the boil over moderate heat. Simmer, partially covered, until the chicken is tender, about 10 minutes. Remove the chicken with a slotted spoon and set aside to cool. Reserve the poaching liquid for the dressing.

Arrange the rinsed lettuce leaves on 4 individual plates. Once the chicken is cool, cut the fillets into thick strips and arrange on the lettuce leaves. Arrange the sliced cucumber on the plates, then slice the nectarines and arrange them on the plates. Arrange 4 baby mealies on each plate.

Heat the reserved poaching liquid in a small saucepan over moderate heat. Mix the cornflour or arrowroot with a little cold water and stir into the poaching liquid. Cook over low heat, stirring, until slightly thickened, about 2 minutes. Remove from the heat and stir in salt and pepper to taste, if needed. Sprinkle the dressing over the chicken and lettuce, crumble the feta cheese over the lettuce and garnish with the parsley sprigs. Serve immediately.
950 kJ per serving

Suitable for: low sodium (use low-salt chicken stock).

Shortcut coronation chicken

(Serves 4-6)

A very much quicker – and healthier – version of the buffet table stalwart.

500 g cold cooked chicken, cut into pieces

CHUTNEY DRESSING
75 ml mango chutney, minus big pieces of fruit
10 ml tomato purée
10 ml medium-strength curry powder
350 g ricotta or smooth cottage cheese
10 ml lemon juice

First make the dressing. Place the chutney, tomato purée and curry powder in a saucepan. Very slowly, bring the mixture to the boil and let it bubble gently for about 2 minutes. Remove from the stove, cool to luke-warm and stir in the ricotta or cottage cheese and lemon juice.
Fold in the chicken, transfer to a bowl and refrigerate, covered, until cold.
Arrange the chicken on a lettuce-lined platter and serve with a rice or pasta salad, or a green salad.
930 kJ per serving

Suitable for: low fat, low cholesterol.

Meat and game

Beef, lamb, mutton, pork and game are all excellent sources of protein, but care has to be taken when choosing beef and lamb cuts, because some of them have a high fat content. Game provides leaner alternatives, and ostrich, for example, can be used to make high-fat dishes such as bobotie and lasagne more acceptable if you have to watch how much fat you consume. If you're on a low-cholesterol diet, watch portion sizes for all meat choices, and combine with other low-cholesterol foods.

BEEF

Choose lean cuts such as fillet, sirloin and rump, and cooking methods that do not require a lot of oil or fat, for the greatest health benefits.

Herbed roast fillet

(Serves 4)

Fillet is a very lean cut, and in this recipe, the quantity of oil called for is just enough to ensure an excellent roast, but not so much that it will play havoc with the fat content.

15 ml extra-virgin olive oil
30 ml mustard powder
600 g beef fillet, sirloin, or silverside

HERB CRUST
1 clove garlic, crushed
30 ml chopped fresh parsley
15 ml chopped fresh chives
15 ml chopped fresh rosemary or tarragon
15 ml coarsely ground black pepper
5-10 ml salt

Combine the olive oil and mustard powder and spread over the meat. Combine all the crust ingredients in a flat dish and roll the meat in the mixture. Tie the beef with lengths of string and transfer to a roasting pan. Set aside for about 30 minutes.
Preheat the oven to 220 °C.
Place the roasting pan in the oven and roast the meat for 15 minutes for a rare roast, or until brown and crusty on the outside and pink and juicy inside. If you prefer your meat well-done, roast the meat for about 20 minutes, or until pale brown inside.
Remove the meat from the oven and leave it to rest in a warm place for about 10 minutes, to allow the juices to settle. Serve hot with baked potatoes and steamed vegetables of your choice, or cold, with salads.
855 kJ per serving

Suitable for: low fat.

Shaved beef salad

(Serves 4)

Just a touch of beef flavour lifts this salad from the ordinary to the extraordinary.

500 g pickling onions
65 ml caster sugar
500 ml balsamic vinegar
1 butter lettuce, separated into leaves
200 g cooked baby beetroot, skinned and left whole
125 g shaved roast beef
3 large mushrooms, wiped and thickly sliced
500 g ripe cherry tomatoes, halved
60 g low-fat mozzarella cheese, chopped
15 ml sesame seeds, toasted
fresh basil leaves to garnish

BASIL DRESSING
60 ml extra-virgin olive oil
25 ml reserved pickling liquid
salt and freshly ground black pepper to taste
15 ml finely chopped fresh basil

Peel the onions and place in a container with an airtight lid. Combine the sugar and vinegar in a saucepan and stir over moderate heat until the sugar has dissolved. Bring to the boil and pour over the onions in the container. Seal while hot and leave overnight.
The next day, remove the onions from the container, using a slotted spoon, and slice. Reserve the pickling liquid.
Arrange the lettuce on 4 individual plates, then arrange the onions, beetroot, shaved beef, mushrooms, tomatoes and cheese on top.
Shake the dressing ingredients together in a jar and drizzle over the salad. Sprinkle toasted sesame seeds on top and serve, garnished with basil leaves.
515 kJ per serving

Suitable for: low gluten, low fat.

Pan-grilled steak

(Serves 4)

Maturing ensures a tender steak, and grilling in a pan brushed with oil cuts down on fats without sacrificing flavour.

4 x 150 g well-matured sirloin or rump steaks, trimmed of all visible fat
extra-virgin olive oil for brushing pan

MARINADE
juice and grated peel of 1 orange
10 ml extra-virgin olive oil
1 clove garlic, crushed
dash Worcestershire sauce
salt and freshly ground black pepper to taste

Mix the marinade ingredients in a large container with a lid. Place the steaks in the container and marinate for at least 6 hours, but preferably overnight. Turn from time to time. Brush a frying pan with a thin layer of oil and heat until very hot. Fry the steaks, one at a time, until cooked to taste. How long the steaks are cooked will depend on how thick they are, a 2 cm thick steak will need about 2 minutes a side for rare, 3-4 minutes a side for medium and 5-6 minutes a side for well-done.
Serve on heated plates, with a plain baked potato and a mixed salad on the side.
1 200 kJ per serving

Suitable for: low fat, low gluten.

Beef and sweet pepper stir-fry

(Serves 4)

Quick to prepare, and a taste beyond compare, make this dish a winner. Use vegetables of your choice to make your stir-fry extra-special.

15 ml extra-virgin olive oil
1 cm piece fresh ginger, peeled and chopped
2 cloves garlic, crushed
4 spring onions, trimmed and thinly sliced
1 red sweet pepper, cored, seeded and thinly sliced

350 g lean steak, trimmed and cut into strips
1 celery stalk, trimmed and thinly sliced
1 carrot, peeled and cut into julienne strips
15 ml dark soy sauce or Worcestershire sauce
salt and freshly ground black pepper to taste

Heat the oil until very hot in a large, heavy-based frying pan. Add the ginger, garlic and spring onions and stir-fry for 2 minutes. Add the sweet pepper and steak and stir-fry for 3 minutes, or until the meat is no longer pink. Add the celery, carrot and soy sauce and stir-fry for 3 minutes. Season to taste and serve at once, with brown rice or bulgur (recipe on page 77).
710 kJ per serving

● High in fibre.

Suitable for: low gluten, low fat.

Veal schnitzel

(Serves 4)

This is the classic veal dish. If veal is unavailable, pork or chicken fillets, beaten until very thin, may be used instead.

4 thin veal fillets (schnitzels)
125 ml flour mixed with 5 ml salt and 2 ml pepper
1 egg, lightly beaten
125 ml breadcrumbs
125 g butter or margarine
lemon slices, sliced hard-boiled egg and rolled anchovy fillets to garnish

Dredge the veal schnitzels in the seasoned flour, dip them in the beaten egg and then in the breadcrumbs, covering completely.
Melt the butter or margarine in a large frying-pan and fry the veal quickly on both sides until golden brown and crisp. Reduce the heat and fry the schnitzels for a few minutes more, to ensure that the veal is cooked. Garnish each schnitzel with a slice of hard-boiled egg topped with a rolled anchovy, and serve with mashed potato and lemon slices on the side.
1 280 kJ per portion

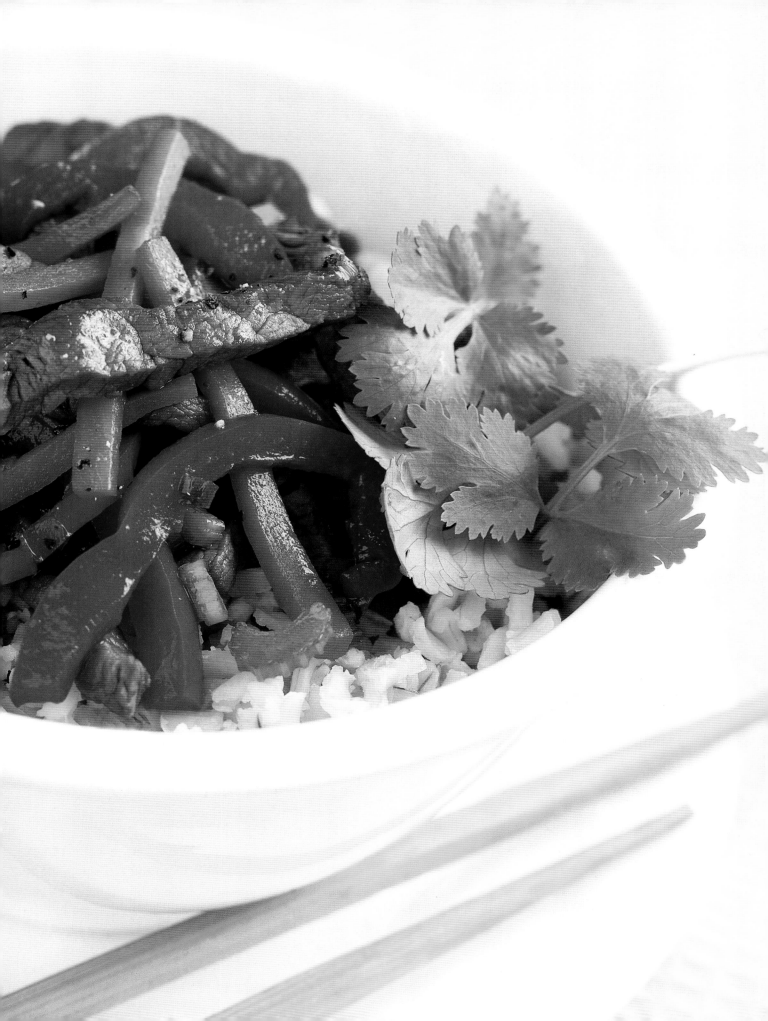

Swiss steak

(Serves 4-6)

This is an excellent recipe for warming up the family on a cold winter's evening. Cooked long and slowly, the steak mince is meltingly tender, and it's even better heated up a day or two later!

canola oil
3 medium leeks, trimmed and sliced
1 kg extra-lean steak mince
salt and freshly ground black pepper to taste

GRAVY
15 ml flour
5 ml chicken stock powder
5 ml gravy powder
10 ml Worcestershire sauce
10 ml balsamic vinegar
45 ml tomato sauce (ketchup) (recipe on page 150)
750 ml water

Heat the oil in a large frying pan. Add the leeks and stir-fry until softened but not browned. Add the mince and brown lightly, stirring from time to time. Remove the mince and leeks from the frying pan, using a slotted spoon to eliminate as much fat as possible, and place in the bowl of a slow cooker.

To make the gravy, place all the ingredients in a saucepan and bring to the boil, stirring from time to time. Boil for 5 minutes, then pour over the mince in the slow cooker. Stir to mix.

Cover with the lid and cook on high for 1 hour, then on low for 2-3 hours, or until the mince is cooked and the flavours are well blended. Serve with rice or mashed potatoes. Season to taste.

950 kJ per serving

● This gravy is an excellent basic one, perfect with many other meat dishes as well.

VARIATIONS
● USE OSTRICH MINCE INSTEAD OF STEAK MINCE.
● USE 1 KG TENDERISED STEAK INSTEAD OF MINCE. DIP IN SEASONED FLOUR, THEN BROWN LIGHTLY ON EITHER SIDE TO SEAL IN THE JUICES. PROCEED AS DESCRIBED IN THE RECIPE.

Suitable for: low fat.

LAMB

These days, lamb is preferred to mutton, even for traditional dishes like tomato bredie, because lamb is tender and less fatty than mutton. It's perfect, too, for kebabs, braaiing and grilling.

Ginger and apricot stuffed lamb

(Serves 8)

A special-occasion roast that most satisfyingly combines piquant and sweet flavours, a combination much loved by many South Africans.

1,5 kg boneless leg or shoulder of lamb

STUFFING
5 ml extra-virgin olive oil
1 small onion, peeled and finely chopped
150 ml coarsely chopped dried apricots
15 ml peeled and grated fresh root ginger
5 ml grated lemon peel
salt and freshly ground black pepper to taste

APRICOT GLAZE
30 ml apricot jam
2 ml prepared mustard
1 ml ground ginger
16 fresh or canned apricot halves, 8 sprigs rosemary or watercress, and 8 fresh or preserved kumquats to garnish

Preheat the oven to 160 °C.

First make the stuffing. Heat the oil in a small saucepan over moderate heat, then add the onion and fry until softened but not browned. Stir in the dried apricots, ginger, lemon peel, and salt and pepper to taste. Place the stuffing in the lamb cavity and sew up to seal. Place the lamb on the rack of a roasting pan and roast for 1½ hours.

To make the glaze, combine the jam, mustard and ginger and mix well. Brush over the outside of the lamb and roast for a further 15 minutes, or until the lamb is brown outside and pink inside. Transfer to a serving platter and allow to stand for 15 minutes before carving. Arrange the apricot halves, rosemary or watercress sprigs and kumquats around the lamb.

1 370 kJ per serving

Suitable for: low gluten, low fat (trim off all visible fat).

Curried lamb kebabs

(Serves 4)

The kebabs may be braaied over the coals instead of grilled in the oven.

500 g lean shoulder of lamb, cut into chunks
coriander sprigs or basil leaves to garnish
50 g toasted flaked almonds

MARINADE
1 green chilli, seeded and sliced
2 cloves garlic, crushed
2 cm piece fresh root ginger, peeled and chopped
15-30 ml curry powder
50 ml low-fat natural yoghurt
30 ml water

Combine all the marinade ingredients. Coat the lamb with marinade and thread onto 8 wooden skewers. Return to the marinade and leave for 1 hour.

Preheat the grill and spray the grilling pan with nonstick cooking spray. Grill the kebabs until cooked through and nicely browned, turning often and basting with the marinade.

Garnish with the coriander or basil leaves and sprinkle the almonds over. Serve immediately.

1 210 kJ per serving

Suitable for: low fat.

Greek kofta kebabs

(Serves 6)

'Meatballs on a stick' combine deliciously with fresh mint and parsley.

500 g lamb or lean steak mince
5 ml ground coriander seeds
5 ml ground cumin seeds
15 ml chopped fresh mint
15 ml chopped fresh parsley or coriander leaves
salt and freshly ground black pepper

Mince or process the lamb or steak mince very finely and combine with remaining ingredients. Shape the mixture into a sausage around thin wooden skewers and place in the freezer for 15-20 minutes to firm slightly. Grill or braai, turning often, for 10 minutes. Serve hot, with noodles and ratatouille (recipe on page 91).

750 kJ per serving

● The kebabs may be made a few hours in advance and refrigerated until ready to grill.

VARIATION: CHILLI POWDER OR TABASCO SAUCE TO TASTE MAY BE ADDED TO THE MINCE FOR SPICIER KEBABS.

Suitable for: low gluten.

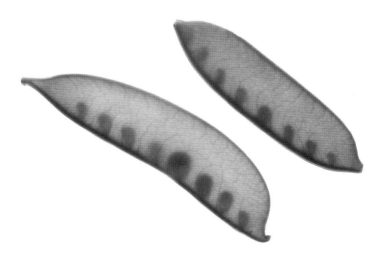

Lamb loin chops with prunes
(Serves 6)

Loin chops are excellent braaied or fried, and they go particularly well with the sweetness of the prunes.

canola oil for frying
6 lamb loin chops
1 large onion, peeled and thinly sliced
10 ml salt
5 ml freshly ground black pepper
18 prunes
150 ml dry red wine
200 ml meat stock
4 whole cloves
2,5 cm piece stick cinnamon
15 ml cornflour

Heat the oil in a large saucepan and brown the chops on both sides over low heat. Pour off all the excess oil, then arrange the onion slices on top of the chops. Sprinkle with salt and pepper. Add the prunes, wine, stock, cloves and cinnamon and simmer, covered, until the chops are tender, about 40 minutes. Add a little more wine or stock if necessary.

Remove the chops and prunes to a heated serving dish and keep them warm. Mix the cornflour with a little water and stir into the sauce in the saucepan. Bring to the boil, then reduce the heat and simmer for 1-2 minutes to thicken, stirring constantly. Spoon the sauce over the chops and serve immediately, with mashed potatoes and steamed vegetables of your choice.
980 kJ per serving

● High in fibre.

VARIATION: USE DRIED NECTARINES OR PEAR HALVES INSTEAD OF THE PRUNES.

Suitable for: low gluten.

Tomato bredie
(Serves 6)

A traditional dish with lasting taste appeal. Using stewing lamb, rather than the usual mutton, reduces the fat content.

25 ml canola oil
2 large onions, peeled and sliced
1 clove garlic, crushed
1 kg stewing lamb, trimmed of visible fat and cut into chunks
10 ml salt
freshly ground black pepper
a little stock, water, or wine
500 g potatoes, peeled and sliced
1 kg tomatoes, skinned and chopped
5 ml sugar
2 ml dried thyme
5 ml dried marjoram

Heat the oil in a large saucepan and sauté the onions and garlic until softened but not browned. Add the meat and brown the cubes quickly on all sides. Add the salt, pepper and a little stock, water or wine and simmer, covered, until the meat starts to get tender. Add the potatoes, tomatoes, sugar, thyme and marjoram and cook for 1 hour longer. Serve with rice, couscous, noodles or crushed wheat.
1 400 kJ per serving

● Using canned tomatoes enhances the flavour.

Suitable for: low gluten.

Spicy lamb curry
(Serves 6)

Lamb makes an excellent curry, especially when the traditional spices are added to sharpen the flavour.

25 ml oil
2 onions, peeled and finely chopped
1 bay leaf
2 ml ground cinnamon

5 ml ground coriander
2 ml ground cumin
2 cloves garlic, crushed
20 ml curry powder
25 ml flour or cornflour
5 ml turmeric
1 kg lamb rib, trimmed of visible fat and cubed
500 g tomatoes, skinned
30 ml fruit chutney
250 ml meat stock
5 ml sugar
salt and freshly ground black pepper to taste

Preheat the oven to 150 °C.
Heat the oil in a large saucepan and sauté the onions until softened but not browned. Add the bay leaf, cinnamon, coriander, cumin, garlic, curry powder, flour and turmeric and simmer for a few minutes, stirring. Add the lamb and a little more oil, if necessary, and brown the meat lightly. Add the remaining ingredients and mix well.
Transfer the mixture to a large casserole dish and bake, covered, for 1½ hours. Serve immediately with boiled rice and various side dishes, including sliced banana, desiccated coconut, diced pineapple and chutney.
1 010 kJ per serving

VARIATION: THE CURRY MAY BE SIMMERED ON TOP OF THE STOVE FOR 1 HOUR, INSTEAD OF BAKING.

Suitable for: low gluten (use cornflour), low fat (make curry ahead of time, leave to cool and skim off all the fat on the surface, then reheat).

PORK
Pork has had a bad press – far from being packed with fat, as it's reputed to be, it is in fact a lean meat because the fat surrounds the meat (and can be cut off), whereas other meats are marbled with fat. In addition, pork is always tender, which makes it really reliable.

Sweet-and-sour pork chops
(Serves 4)

Fresh cubed pineapple may be used instead of marmalade to achieve the sweet-and-sour result.

4 pork loin chops, trimmed of fat
30 ml orange marmalade
30 ml light soy sauce
10 ml prepared coarse-grained mustard
1 chilli, seeded and diced
3 ml grated fresh root ginger
75 ml cold water
15 ml cornflour
4 spring onions, trimmed and chopped
freshly ground black pepper

Spray a nonstick frying pan lightly with nonstick cooking spray. Add the chops and pan-grill for 5 minutes, then turn them over.
Combine the marmalade, soy sauce, mustard, chilli, ginger and water in a bowl and pour over the chops. Cover and cook for 10-15 minutes, or until the chops are done.
Blend the cornflour with 30 ml cold water to form a smooth paste. Stir into the liquid in the pan and heat until the sauce thickens.
Serve on cooked noodles or couscous, garnished with spring onions and freshly ground black pepper.
1 360 kJ per serving

VARIATIONS
- TWO PORK FILLETS MAY BE USED INSTEAD OF THE CHOPS.
- TO REDUCE THE NUMBER OF KILOJOULES, USE A LOW-SUGAR MARMALADE OR FRUIT PURÉE.

Suitable for: low gluten, low fat.

Gingered pork stir-fry

(Serves 4)

Cider in the marinade adds a sweetish flavour to the stir-fry.

500 g pork fillet, cut into thin strips
10 ml canola oil
2,5 cm piece fresh root ginger, peeled and chopped
1 bunch spring onions, trimmed and sliced
1 green, 1 yellow and 1 red sweet pepper, cored, seeded and sliced
5 ml cornflour
15 ml light soy sauce

MARINADE
150 ml dry cider (Savanna)
5 ml mustard powder
1 clove garlic, crushed
coarsely ground black pepper to taste
5 ml soy sauce

Combine the marinade ingredients, add the meat and stir to coat well. Marinate, in the refrigerator, for 1-2 hours. Remove the meat from the marinade.
Heat the oil in a large, heavy-based frying pan and add the pork and ginger. Stir-fry over high heat for 2-3 minutes.
Add the spring onions and peppers, and stir-fry for 3 minutes.
In a small bowl, blend the cornflour with the marinade and soy sauce. Add to the meat mixture. Bring quickly to the boil and cook until thick and glossy. Serve immediately on a bed of noodles or brown rice.
995 kJ per serving

● High in fibre.

VARIATION: ADD 1 RED APPLE, CORED AND SLICED, TO THE STIR-FRY TO EXTEND THE FLAVOUR OF THE CIDER.

Suitable for: low fat, low gluten (omit the noodles, or use rice noodles).

Pork fillet with apple crust

(Serves 4)

Apple and pork go well together, and the apple in this recipe imparts a marvellous flavour to the meat.

500 g lean pork fillet
5 ml salt
coarsely ground black pepper to taste
450 g can unsweetened pie apple
½ onion, peeled and finely chopped
1 cm piece fresh root ginger, peeled and chopped
15 ml brown sugar
125 ml dried breadcrumbs

Preheat the oven to 220 °C.
Season the meat with salt and pepper. Combine the apple, onion, ginger and brown sugar in a bowl.
Place the pork in a roasting pan and spread the apple mixture over the meat. Sprinkle the breadcrumbs over. Roast the pork fillet for about 30 minutes, or until just done. Remove from the oven and set aside in a warm place for 5 minutes.
Carve the pork on the diagonal and serve hot, with the apple mixture and brown rice or crushed wheat.
1 025 kJ per serving

VARIATION: USE STEWED APRICOTS OR PEACHES INSTEAD OF THE APPLES AND MIX THE BREAD-CRUMBS WITH A LITTLE GROUND CINNAMON.

Suitable for: low fat, low gluten (omit the breadcrumbs).

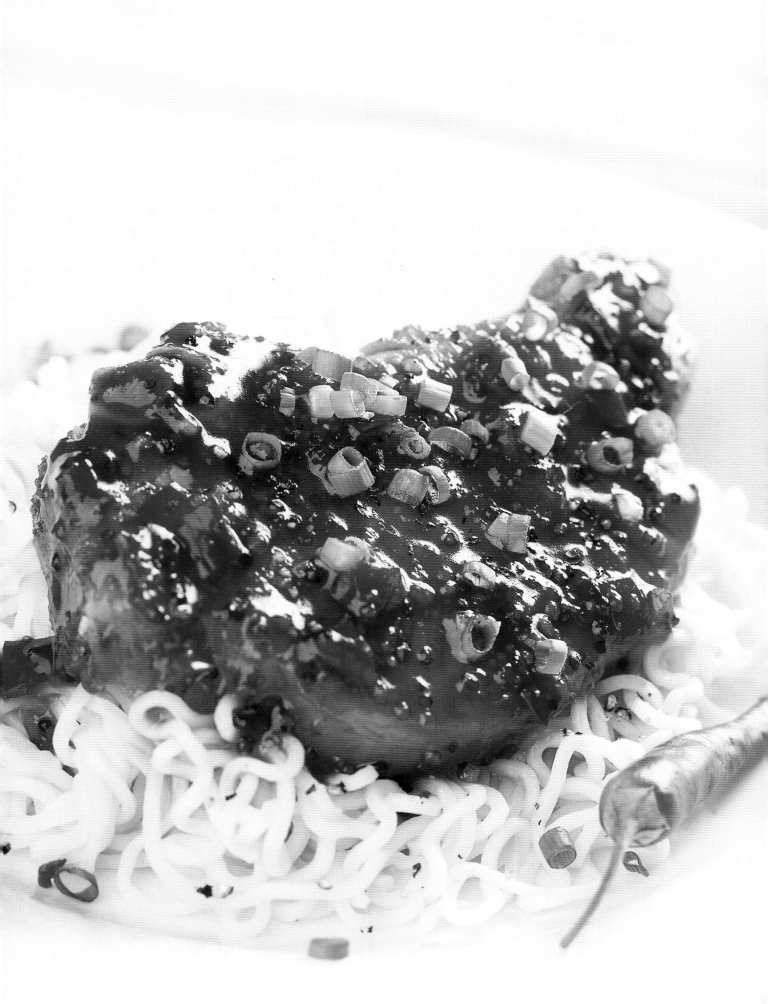

Paprika pork

(Serves 4)

This simplified version of the Hungarian dish takes far less time to prepare, but it's every bit as tasty. Add red sweet pepper strips to enhance the flavour, if you wish.

30 ml canola oil
3 onions, peeled and thinly sliced
600 g pork fillet, cut into chunks
30 ml paprika
300 ml vegetable stock or low-salt chicken stock (recipe on page 149)
100 ml crème fraîche or low-fat creamed cottage cheese
fresh chives to garnish

Heat the oil in a saucepan, add the onions and fry until softened, but not browned. Add the pork to the pan and brown over fairly high heat. Stir in the paprika and stir-fry for 1 minute, then add stock and bring to the boil.
Cover the saucepan with the lid and cook over moderate heat until the pork is tender, about 25 minutes. Stir in the crème fraîche or low-fat creamed cottage cheese and simmer for a further 2 minutes.
Transfer to a serving dish, snip chives over and serve immediately with brown rice and steamed broccoli.
1 500 kJ per serving

Suitable for: low fat, low gluten.

Herbed pork fillet roast

(Serves 4)

It's the easiest roast ever, and among the best-tasting, because the meat flavours the vegetables as they cook.

4 medium parsnips, peeled and quartered lengthways
600 g butternut, peeled, seeded and cut into chunks
2 onions, peeled and cut into wedges
15 ml extra-virgin olive oil
salt and freshly ground black pepper to taste
grated peel of 1 lemon or lime

10 ml dried Italian herbs
500 g pork fillet
1 medium Granny Smith apple, peeled, cored and cut into chunks
400 ml hot chicken stock or low-salt chicken stock (recipe on page 149)

Preheat the oven to 200 °C.
Place the vegetables in a roasting pan, drizzle with olive oil, season and toss together.
Mix the lemon peel with the Italian herbs and roll the pork fillet in the mixture. Place on top of the vegetables. Roast for 40 minutes.
Scatter the apple pieces over the vegetables, then add the hot stock and cook for a further 15-20 minutes.
Remove the meat from the oven and allow to stand, lightly covered, for a few minutes. Slice the pork, arrange on a platter with the vegetables and sprinkle a little of the pan juices on top. Serve with rice or noodles.
1 650 kJ per serving

● High in fibre.

Suitable for: low fat, low gluten.

GAME

All kinds of game meat are the perfect lean choice. Ostrich, in particular, has gained in popularity both in South Africa and other parts of the world – which accounts for its rise to gourmet status (and prices)! It's a well-earned popularity, because ostrich is an excellent alternative to fattier meat cuts and makes it possible for those watching kilojoule and fat intake to enjoy many dishes that would otherwise be taboo.

Braised ostrich

(Serves 6)

An excellent dish if you are watching the kilojoules, and it's rich in fibre too!

1 kg ostrich steak
1 litre low-fat natural yoghurt
25 ml extra-virgin olive oil

2 cloves garlic, chopped
1 onion, peeled and sliced
1 green sweet pepper, cored, seeded and sliced
2 stalks celery, trimmed and chopped
1 leek, trimmed and sliced
500 ml meat stock, low-salt chicken stock (recipe
    on page 149), or water
250 ml dry red wine
10 ml salt (omit if stock is used)
5 ml chopped fresh thyme
freshly ground black pepper
10 ml flour
400 g button mushrooms
100 g dried peaches, chopped

Place the meat in a container, pour the yoghurt over and marinate for 2 days in the refrigerator. Cube the meat and discard the marinade.

Heat the oil in a large frying pan and sauté the garlic, onion, green pepper, celery and leek until softened but not browned. Add the meat and brown lightly. Add the stock or water, wine, salt (if using), thyme and pepper. Cover and simmer over low heat for 1 hour. Thicken the gravy with the flour mixed to a paste with a little of the pan juices, then add the mushrooms and peaches and simmer for a further 10 minutes. Serve with crushed wheat or brown rice.

900 kJ per serving

Suitable for: low cholesterol, low fat, low gluten, low salt (omit salt and use low-salt chicken stock).

Ostrich bobotie
(Serves 8)

The traditional dish uses lean minced beef, but ostrich mince makes an excellent substitute – it's lean, tender and combines very well with the other ingredients during cooking.

1 slice white bread
125 ml milk
1 kg ostrich mince
1 medium-sized onion, peeled and finely chopped
125 ml seedless raisins (optional)

125 ml blanched almonds (optional)
15 ml apricot jam
15 ml fruit chutney
10 ml salt
2 ml pepper
10 ml butter or canola oil

TOPPING
3 eggs
125 ml milk
25 ml lemon juice
10 ml curry powder
5 ml turmeric
5 ml salt
2 lemon or bay leaves

Preheat the oven to 180 °C.

Soak the bread in milk, squeeze to remove the excess milk (reserve milk for topping) and mix the bread with the ostrich mince. Mix in all the other ingredients, except the butter or oil, and the topping ingredients.

Melt the butter or heat the oil in a frying pan and brown the meat mixture lightly in it. Turn out into an ovenproof dish.

To make the topping, beat the eggs, milk, lemon juice, curry powder, turmeric and salt together and pour over the meat. Garnish with the lemon or bay leaves.

Bake until set, about 50 minutes. Serve with white or yellow rice.

1 200 kJ per serving

● Bobotie freezes very well.

Suitable for: low fat.

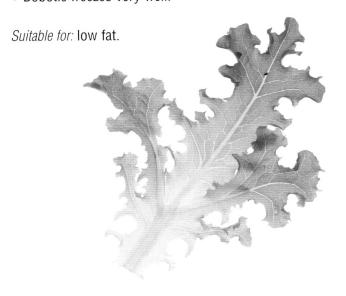

Pan-grilled venison steaks in wine sauce

(Serves 8)

Any tender venison cut may be used in this recipe.

5-10 ml salt
8 tender venison steaks
25 ml extra-virgin olive oil or canola oil
1 onion, peeled and chopped
250 g mushrooms, wiped clean and sliced
100 ml red wine
5 ml Worcestershire sauce
250 ml low-fat natural yoghurt
25 ml flour
5 ml chopped fresh thyme
freshly ground black pepper to taste

Sprinkle salt over the steaks. Heat the oil in a frying pan and sauté the onion and mushrooms until softened but not overcooked. Remove from the pan and keep warm. Heat the frying pan to very hot and pan-grill the steaks on both sides until just done, 2-3 minutes a side.
Return the onion and mushrooms to the pan and add the wine and Worcestershire sauce. Bring to the boil. Meanwhile, combine the yoghurt with the flour and pour over the meat. Stir in the thyme and black pepper and simmer for 5 minutes, until slightly thickened. Serve immediately, with brown rice or noodles.
910 kJ per serving

Suitable for: low fat.

Springbok potjiekos

(Serves 8)

If you thought potjiekos was a thing of the past, try this lean cuisine version.

25 ml canola oil
4 carrots, peeled and sliced
2 onions, peeled and sliced
2 cloves garlic, crushed
10 ml chopped fresh thyme or sage
1 kg springbok meat, cubed

250 g bacon, chopped (optional)
500 ml port or dry red wine
6 potatoes, peeled and sliced

Heat the oil in a cast-iron pot over the coals and sauté the carrots, onions and garlic until softened but not overcooked. Add the thyme or sage, venison, bacon (if using) and port or red wine. Simmer, covered, over the coals for 3 hours. Add the potatoes and simmer for a further 30-45 minutes. Serve with mealie meal porridge.
1 010 kJ per serving

● High in fibre.

Suitable for: low fat (omit the bacon), low gluten.

Fish and seafood

Fish is a marvellous food, because it provides protein and other nutrients without adding too much extra fat – as long as the cooking method doesn't use too much fat or oil. Grilling, baking, dry-pan grilling, braaiing, steaming and poaching offer a variety of cooking methods that won't pile on the kilojoules, and most fish cook really well in the microwave oven, providing results that are tender and moist.

Snoek over the coals

(Serves 8-10)

No other fish can quite match the flavour of snoek, especially if it is cooked over the coals. It's an oily fish, so this cooking method is excellent for removing the excess oil and ensuring a delectable result.

1 whole fresh snoek, entrails removed
melted butter, margarine, or olive oil
15 ml salt
5 ml coarsely ground pepper
lemon juice

Wash the snoek well. Brush the outside with melted butter, margarine, or olive oil. Season, inside and out,

with salt and pepper and sprinkle a little lemon juice inside. Wrap the snoek securely in a large sheet of greased foil and cook under the grill or over hot coals until the fish is tender, 30-40 minutes. Serve hot.
675 kJ per serving

VARIATION: THE SNOEK MAY BE GRILLED WITHOUT WRAPPING, BUT REMEMBER TO BRUSH IT FREQUENTLY WITH MELTED BUTTER WHILE IT IS COOKING.

Suitable for: low gluten, low sodium (use herbs instead of salt), low cholesterol (use olive oil).

Smoorsnoek
(Serves 6)

No West Coast meal would be complete without smoorsnoek served on rice, with a few sambals on the side.

1 kg cooked snoek, skin and bones removed
25 ml oil
1 large onion, peeled and chopped
2 cloves garlic, crushed
2 large potatoes, peeled and thinly sliced, or cubed cooked potatoes
2 medium tomatoes, skinned and quartered
1 small green sweet pepper, cored, seeded and chopped
5 ml salt
2 ml freshly ground black pepper

Flake the fish. Heat the oil in a saucepan and sauté the onion and garlic until transparent. Add the potatoes and sauté until they start to soften, stirring often. Add the tomatoes, green pepper and flaked snoek, shake to mix well and simmer until the fish is heated through. Season and mix well. Serve on a bed of rice, accompanied by a fresh green salad.
885 kJ per serving
● High in fibre.

VARIATIONS
● USE SMOKED SNOEK, OR A COMBINATION OF FRESH AND SMOKED SNOEK, INSTEAD OF THE FRESH FISH.
● USE SALTED SNOEK INSTEAD OF FRESH SNOEK. SOAK IN COLD WATER FOR 1 HOUR, THEN DRAIN AND COOK IN FRESH WATER. DO NOT ADD EXTRA SALT.

Suitable for: low gluten, low cholesterol.

Pickled fish
(Serves 8-10)

In years gone by, no picnic or summer lunch was complete without a big dish of pickled fish to enjoy with salads and bread.

2,5 kg Cape salmon, kingklip, yellowtail or any other firm-fleshed white fish
4 onions, peeled and sliced
750 ml vinegar
125 ml water
20 ml salt
125 ml sugar
30 ml curry powder
turmeric to taste
2 ml cayenne pepper
1 piece fresh root ginger, crushed
10 coriander seeds
5 lemon or bay leaves

Clean and fillet the fish and cut it into portions. Combine all the other ingredients in a deep saucepan and simmer for 20 minutes. Carefully add the fish and simmer for a further 20 minutes. Take care not to break the fish.
Remove the fish with a slotted spoon and layer the portions in a glass or stainless steel dish. Pour the curry sauce over. Leave to cool, then cover tightly and store for 2-3 days before use.
850 kJ per serving

Suitable for: low cholesterol, low gluten.

Fish bobotie

(Serves 6)

Another traditional favourite. Any firm-fleshed white fish may be used.

500 g cooked white fish, skinned and boned
1 thick slice white bread, crusts removed
300 ml low-fat milk
25 ml canola oil
1 large onion, peeled and coarsely chopped
juice of 1 lemon
10 ml curry powder
25 ml seedless raisins
25 ml chopped blanched almonds
5 ml salt
1 ml freshly ground black pepper
2 large eggs
2 bay or lemon leaves

Preheat the oven to 180 °C.
Flake the fish and place in a bowl. Soak the bread in the milk. Heat the oil in a frying pan and sauté the onion until transparent. Add the lemon juice, curry powder, raisins, almonds, salt and pepper and cook for 1 minute. Add the fish. Squeeze the excess milk from the bread and set it aside. Mix the bread and fish thoroughly.
Beat the eggs, add the reserved milk and beat the mixture again until well blended.
Place the fish mixture in a greased ovenproof dish. Pour the egg and milk mixture over and top with the bay or lemon leaves.
Bake until set, about 35 minutes. Serve hot, with boiled rice, desiccated coconut and fruit chutney.
620 kJ per serving

Steenbras kebabs

(Serves 6)

Fish threaded onto skewers and then cooked in the oven or over the coals is a dish found in virtually every cuisine in the world. What adds a different flavour here is the particularly succulent fish.

1,5 kg steenbras, skinned, filleted and cubed
6 bay leaves or lemon leaves, halved
6 cherry tomatoes
12 brown mushroom caps

MARINADE
6 thick wedges onion
juice of 1 lemon
10 ml wine vinegar
250 ml canola oil
1 ml each dried thyme, basil and rosemary
7 ml salt
2 ml freshly ground black pepper

Preheat the oven to 200 °C.
Combine all the marinade ingredients in a bowl. Add the pieces of fish and the bay or lemon leaves and marinate for 30 minutes. Remove the fish from the marinade, drain on absorbent paper and reserve the marinade.
Thread the ingredients onto 6 skewers in the following order: tomato, fish, ½ bay leaf (or lemon leaf), fish, onion, fish, mushroom cap.
Place the skewers in a greased shallow ovenproof dish. Spoon 25 ml of the marinade over the kebabs and cover the dish with foil, dull side out. Bake for 10 minutes. Remove from the oven.
Preheat the grill. Remove the foil and place the kebabs under the grill. Grill on all sides until cooked, basting frequently with the marinade.
Remove from the grill, add more salt and pepper if necessary and serve immediately with a salad.
1 000 kJ per serving

VARIATIONS
- INSTEAD OF BAKING THE KEBABS, BRAAI THEM OVER THE COALS, ABOUT 300 MM ABOVE THE HEAT, FOR 10 MINUTES. BASTE AND TURN THE KEBABS OFTEN TO ENSURE THAT THEY COOK EVENLY.
- ANY FIRM-FLESHED FISH MAY BE USED INSTEAD OF STEENBRAS.

Suitable for: low gluten, low fat, low cholesterol.

Sole Florentine

(Serves 4)

The flavour of sole goes particularly well with spinach. Choose large East Coast soles, if you can find them.

4 large, or 8 small, sole fillets (625 g in total)
1 onion, peeled and chopped
½ bay leaf
30 ml lemon juice
3 whole peppercorns
2 ml salt
175 ml dry white wine
500 g fresh spinach, ribs discarded
20 ml butter or margarine
25 ml all-purpose flour or arrowroot
125 ml low-fat milk
salt and freshly ground black pepper to taste
15 ml grated Parmesan cheese

Preheat the oven to 180 °C.
Roll up the sole fillets and secure them with toothpicks. Arrange the fillets in a saucepan just large enough to hold them in a single layer. Add the onion, bay leaf, lemon juice, peppercorns and salt. Pour in the wine. Bring to the boil, then cover, reduce the heat, and simmer for 5 minutes. Remove the fillets from the poaching liquid, and reserve the liquid.
Wash the spinach and cook, covered, in just the water clinging to the leaves. Drain and squeeze out the excess water. Chop finely.
Place the spinach in a shallow greased dish just large enough to hold the fish rolls. Place the fish on top.
Strain the reserved poaching liquid and measure off 250 ml (add water, if necessary). Melt the butter in a small saucepan, remove from the stove and stir in the flour until combined. Return to the stove and whisk in the poaching liquid, milk and salt and pepper to taste. Bring to the boil, stirring constantly. Remove from the heat.
Pour the sauce over the fish and sprinkle with the Parmesan cheese. Bake for 10-20 minutes, or until the sauce bubbles.
950 kJ per serving

Suitable for: low cholesterol (use margarine).

Steamed kabeljou

(Serves 6-8)

Fish steamed in a bamboo steamer is a firm favourite in the East; on the east coast of South Africa you may find fish steamed in banana leaves.

2 kg whole kabeljou, or any other firm-fleshed
white fish, scaled and gutted but left whole
10 ml salt
5 ml freshly squeezed lemon juice

Sprinkle the cleaned fish with the salt and lemon juice. Half-fill the bottom of a fish steamer with boiling water (or use a saucepan large enough to support a plate or suspend a wire basket above the water).
Place the fish on the plate or in the wire basket, first wrapping in foil if desired.
Cover tightly with the lid and allow the water to boil briskly so that the fish is enveloped in steam. Steam until done, 10-20 minutes. To test whether the fish is ready, prick it with a fork; if done, the flesh will flake easily.
Steamed fish can be served either plain or with the sauce of your choice.
820 kJ per serving

Suitable for: low fat, low cholesterol, low sodium (omit salt), low gluten.

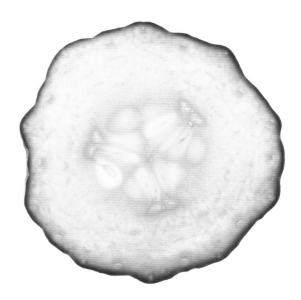

Poached salmon trout with stir-fried ratatouille

(Serves 4)

Salmon trout has a flavour and colour very similar to that of Scottish or Norwegian salmon, and poaching is a particularly good way of preparing it. The stir-fried vegetables add a robust flavour to the dish.

4 x 200 g salmon trout fillets

POACHING LIQUID
1 onion, peeled and chopped
½ bay leaf
30 ml lemon juice
3 whole peppercorns
2 ml salt
200 ml fruity rosé or blanc de noir wine

STIR-FRIED RATATOUILLE
20 ml canola or olive oil
1 small onion, peeled and sliced
2 cloves garlic, crushed
6 medium mushrooms, wiped and halved
1 small yellow or red sweet pepper, cored, seeded and cubed
250 ml cubed brinjals (unpeeled)
1 small baby marrow, trimmed and sliced
2 firm, ripe tomatoes, cut into wedges
2 ml each dried thyme and basil
salt and freshly ground pepper to taste

Combine the poaching liquid ingredients in a saucepan just large enough to hold the fish in a single layer, and bring to the boil. Reduce the heat and carefully add the salmon trout fillets. The poaching liquid should just cover the fish. Simmer, covered, for 10-15 minutes, or until the fish has turned pale pink and flakes easily. Remove the fish from the saucepan and keep warm in the oven.
RATATOUILLE: Make the ratatouille while the fish is cooking. Heat half the oil in a large nonstick frying pan over medium-high heat. Add the onion, garlic, mushrooms and sweet pepper and stir-fry until tender, about 4 minutes. Remove the vegetables to a side dish, using a slotted spoon, and set aside.

Heat the remaining oil in the frying pan and add the brinjals and baby marrow. Stir-fry for 4 minutes, or until tender. Return the mushroom mixture to the pan, then add the tomatoes, thyme and basil. Cover and simmer for 5 minutes. Season to taste and serve with the salmon trout.
850 kJ per serving (fish)
450 kJ per serving (ratatouille)

● High in fibre.

VARIATION: THE POACHING LIQUID MAY BE USED TO MAKE A SAUCE FOR THE SALMON, IF DESIRED.

Suitable for: low cholesterol.

Grilled angelfish with warm mushroom and watercress salad

(Serves 4)

Angelfish is a very tasty fish, which goes particularly well with the flavour of peppers and mushrooms.

1 angelfish, filleted and cut into 4 portions
canola oil for brushing
salt and freshly ground black pepper to taste

SALAD
125 ml extra-virgin olive oil
65 ml water
75 ml lemon juice
2 ml caster sugar
1 small red sweet pepper, cored, seeded and finely chopped
30 ml chopped fresh oregano
250 g button mushrooms
1 small radicchio
375 ml watercress sprigs

First make the salad. Combine the oil, water, lemon juice, sugar, sweet pepper and oregano in a large bowl. Stir in the mushrooms, cover and refrigerate overnight. Next day, transfer the mixture to a saucepan and stir over low heat without boiling until heated through, about 8 minutes.
While the salad is being heated, prepare the fish. Preheat

the grill. Brush the angelfish fillets with oil and season lightly with salt and pepper. Grill the fish for about 2 minutes on either side, or until opaque and the flesh flakes easily when tested with a fork.

Place the salad mixture in a large bowl and add the radicchio and watercress. Toss and serve with the grilled angelfish.

750 kJ per serving

● High in fibre.

To cook in the microwave: Microwave the mushroom mixture for the salad on 100% power for about 2 minutes, or until heated through. Continue as described in the recipe.

Suitable for: low sodium (omit salt).

Smoked haddock crumble

(Serves 4)

This is a delicious way to prepare smoked haddock, and the perfect family supper.

500 g smoked haddock fillets
cold water
15 ml cornflour or arrowroot
300 ml cold low-fat milk
5 ml prepared English mustard
15 ml dried whole-wheat breadcrumbs

CRUMBLE
75 g half-fat Cheddar cheese, grated
15 ml dried whole-wheat breadcrumbs

Soak the haddock for 10 minutes in cold water, changing the water twice to reduce saltiness. Drain and flake the fish.

Preheat the oven to 220 °C.

Tip the cornflour into a saucepan and blend until smooth with a little cold milk. Whisk in the remaining milk and cook over low heat, stirring, until the sauce starts to boil and thicken. Reduce the heat and simmer for 2 minutes, then remove from the stove. Add the fish and mustard and stir in the crumbs.

Spoon the mixture into a lightly greased 1 litre pie dish,

spread it out evenly with a knife and sprinkle the cheese and crumbs over.

Bake for 10-15 minutes, or until browned and bubbly. Serve piping hot with steamed vegetables of your choice, or a mixed salad.

1 030 kJ per serving

Suitable for: low cholesterol (use low-fat cheese for crumble).

Baked pilchard fish cakes in tomato sauce

(Serves 4)

This is a really easy dish to make, and it tastes marvellous.

1 x 425 g can pilchards in tomato sauce, drained
1 small onion, peeled and grated
1 thick slice whole-wheat bread, soaked in water
  and squeezed dry
1 egg
10 ml chopped fresh parsley
salt and freshly ground black pepper to taste

SAUCE
1 large ripe tomato, peeled and chopped
pinch dried Italian herbs
65 ml tomato cocktail, mixed with 15 ml flour
reserved canning liquid

Preheat the oven to 180 °C.

Mash the pilchards and mix with the onion, bread, egg and parsley. Season to taste. Shape the mixture into balls and place them next to one another in a greased ovenproof dish.

Mix all the sauce ingredients together well and pour over the fish cakes in the dish. Bake for 30-45 minutes, or until the fish cakes are cooked and the sauce is bubbling.

Serve with mashed potatoes and peas.

935 kJ per serving

● High in fibre.

Suitable for: low cholesterol.

Microwave fish Provençale

(Serves 4)

Tomatoes and onions go really well with white fish, and cooking in the microwave locks in all the flavours.

1 x 400 g can tomatoes
500 g fresh or frozen white fish fillets
salt and freshly ground black pepper
50 ml chopped fresh parsley
50 ml fine fresh breadcrumbs
25 ml minced spring onions, including tops
15 ml butter, melted
2 cloves garlic, minced

Drain and coarsely chop the tomatoes. Spoon half the tomatoes into a microwave dish just large enough to hold the fish in a single layer. Arrange the fish on top, sprinkle with salt and pepper and top with the remaining tomatoes.
In a small bowl, combine the parsley, breadcrumbs, onions, butter and garlic. Sprinkle over the tomatoes. Partially cover the dish and microwave on 100% power for 9-12 minutes, or until the fish is opaque. Let stand for 3 minutes before serving.
950 kJ per serving

To cook conventionally: Bake at 230 °C for 20 minutes (fresh fish), or 40 minutes (frozen fish).

Suitable for: low cholesterol, low fat.

Kingklip and spinach stir-fry with spring onions

(Serves 4)

Any firm-fleshed white fish may be used instead of the kingklip.

500 g kingklip fillets
30 ml olive or canola oil
1 clove garlic, crushed
10 ml chopped fresh tarragon or 5 ml dried
5 spring onions, thinly sliced
500 g baby spinach leaves
65 ml unsalted cashews
50 ml dry white vermouth (optional)
salt and freshly ground black pepper

Cut the kingklip fillets into thin strips. Heat the oil in a wok or a large heavy-based frying pan and stir-fry the garlic, tarragon and spring onions for 1 minute. Add the fish and stir-fry until opaque, about 3 minutes. Add the spinach and nuts, and stir-fry for 1 minute. Add the vermouth (if using) and cook, covered, for 1 minute. Season, if necessary, and serve hot with noodles.
785 kJ per serving

Suitable for: low gluten, low cholesterol (omit nuts).

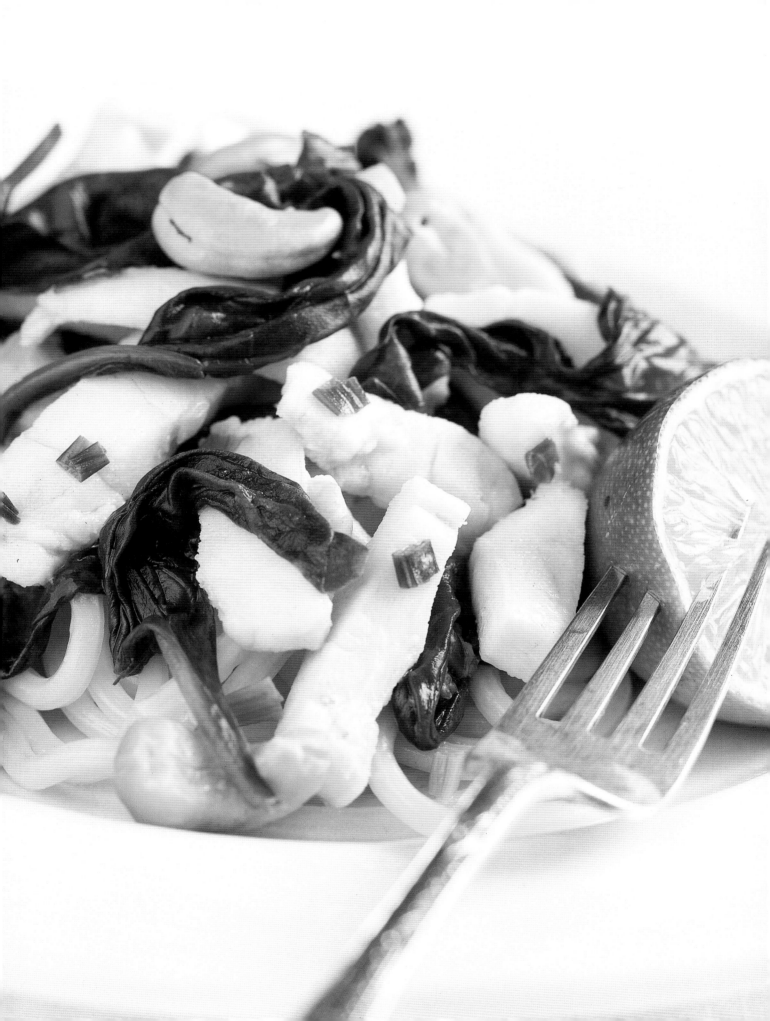

Yellowtail with yoghurt and green pea sauce

(Serves 4)

Dry-frying an oily fish like yellowtail adds to the flavour and cuts down on the quantity of fats it contains.

15 ml canola oil
salt and freshly ground black pepper to taste
4 x 175 g yellowtail fillets

SAUCE
30 ml canola oil
1 ml cumin seeds
300 g frozen petits pois
pinch of sugar
pinch of salt
45 ml desiccated coconut
75 ml low-fat natural yoghurt

First make the sauce. Heat the oil in a wok or heavy-based frying pan and add the cumin seeds. As they darken, stir in the peas. Add a little water, the sugar and salt and cook, uncovered, until the peas are soft. Remove from the heat and stir in the coconut.

Brush a heavy-based saucepan with oil and heat until very hot. Season the fish on both sides. Place the fish in the pan and fry on each side for 3-4 minutes, or until done and it flakes easily.

Stir the yoghurt into the warm peas and adjust the seasoning, if necessary. Serve with the yellowtail and minted new potatoes.

1 900 kJ per serving

VARIATION: USE SALMON TROUT INSTEAD OF YELLOWTAIL.

Suitable for: low cholesterol (omit coconut), low gluten.

Baked kabeljou en papillote

(Serves 4)

Kingklip, salmon trout and yellowtail are equally good prepared this way.

30 ml olive oil
1 carrot, peeled and cut into strips
1 red sweet pepper, cored, seeded and cut into strips
1 clove garlic, chopped
thinly pared peel of 1 lemon, cut into thin strips
freshly squeezed juice of 1 lemon
15 ml chopped fresh chives
5 ml salt
freshly ground black pepper to taste
4 kabeljou fillets
50 ml off-dry white wine or apple juice

Preheat the oven to 180 °C.

Heat the oil in a frying pan and add the carrot, sweet pepper, garlic, lemon peel and juice, and chives, and stir-fry until softened. Sprinkle with salt and pepper to taste. Place each piece of fish on a large piece of non-stick baking parchment. Spoon the topping over, and sprinkle over the wine or apple juice.

Fold into parcels and place on a baking sheet. Bake for 15 minutes, then unwrap and serve with boiled new potatoes.

700 kJ per serving

● High in fibre.

Suitable for: low fat, low cholesterol, low gluten.

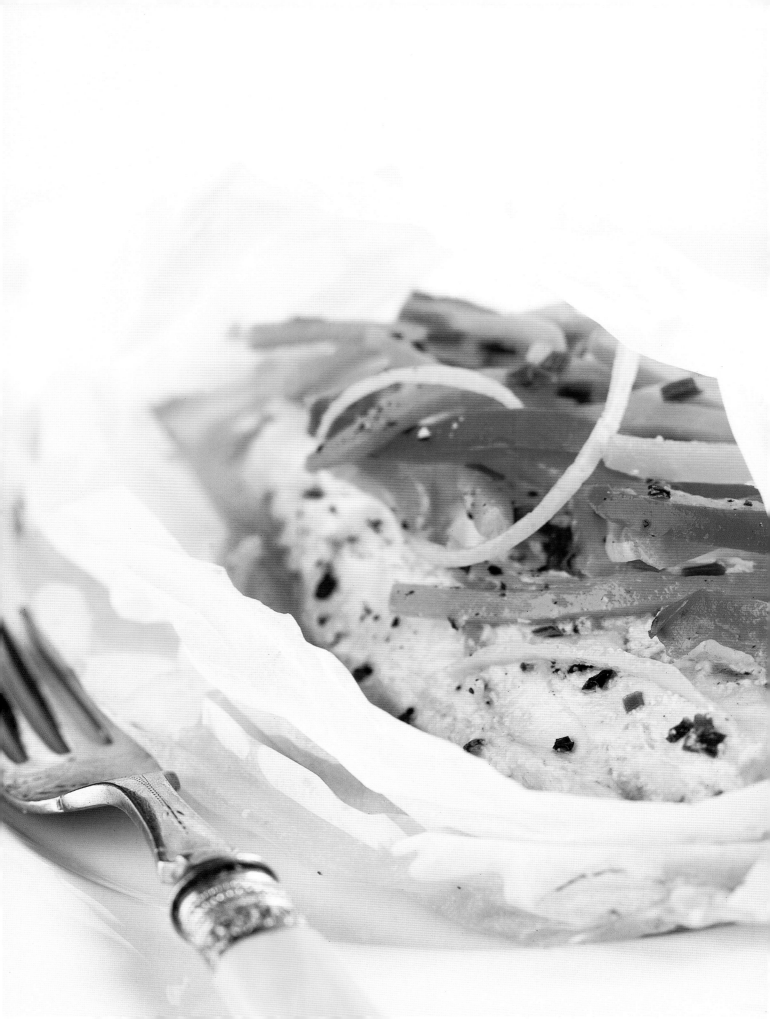

Fish puffs with yoghurt hollandaise

(Serves 4)

These little soufflés have a piquant taste that goes particularly well with the low-fat hollandaise sauce.

65 ml dried breadcrumbs
250 g white fish fillets, chopped
125 ml stale white breadcrumbs
85 ml low-fat smooth cottage cheese
2 ml Tabasco sauce
5 ml grated lemon peel
30 ml chopped fresh chives
2 eggs, separated, plus 2 egg whites
30 ml grated Parmesan cheese
yoghurt hollandaise (recipe on page 150)

Preheat the oven to 190 °C.
Grease 4 x 125 ml soufflé dishes. Sprinkle the insides with dried breadcrumbs and shake away the excess.
Purée the fish until smooth, then add the stale breadcrumbs, cottage cheese, Tabasco sauce, lemon peel, chives and egg yolks and process until combined. Transfer to a large bowl.
Whisk all the egg whites until stiff peaks form, and fold them into the fish mixture. Spoon the mixture evenly into the prepared dishes and sprinkle with cheese. Bake for about 20 minutes or until puffed up and golden. Serve immediately, with yoghurt hollandaise.
670 kJ per serving

Mussels with tomato

(Serves 2)

Eat with a fork and spoon; the fork to pull the mussels out of their shells, the spoon to consume the heavenly broth. The quantities may be doubled, to serve 4.

5 ml olive oil
1 small onion, peeled and finely chopped
1 clove garlic, crushed
pinch each dried thyme and oregano
2 fresh ripe tomatoes, coarsely chopped
50 ml dry white wine

1 kg fresh mussels in their shells, scrubbed and beards removed
50 ml chopped fresh parsley

Heat the oil in a large, heavy-based saucepan over moderate heat. Add the onion and garlic and cook for 2-3 minutes, or until transparent. Stir in the thyme and oregano, then add the tomatoes, breaking them up with the back of a spoon. Bring to the boil and boil for about 2 minutes, uncovered, to reduce the quantity of liquid. Add the wine and return to the boil.
Add the mussels, cover the saucepan and steam for 5 minutes, or until the shells open and the mussels are cooked. Discard any shells that don't open. Sprinkle with parsley. Ladle the mussels into large soup bowls, and spoon the tomato mixture over them. Serve with chunky Italian bread.
720 kJ per serving

Suitable for: low gluten.

Marinated seafood salad

(Serves 4)

Crab sticks may be used if crayfish is unavailable.

500 g cooked hake fillets, cut into strips
1 green sweet pepper, cored, seeded and cut into strips
½ Chinese cabbage, shredded
200 ml sugar snap peas (optional)
8 cherry tomatoes, halved
2 onions, peeled and cut into eighths
250 ml bean sprouts
3 carrots, peeled and cut into strips
375 ml cooked crayfish chunks

MARINADE
75 ml fresh lime or lemon juice
10 ml sunflower oil
2 ml sesame oil (optional)
6 slices fresh ginger

DRESSING
75 ml fresh lime or lemon juice
30 ml sunflower oil

1 clove garlic, crushed
15 ml soy sauce
5 ml chilli sauce (optional)
5 ml brown sugar

Combine the marinade ingredients and marinate the fish strips in it overnight in the refrigerator. Drain and discard the marinade. Combine the fish with the vegetables and crayfish in a large salad bowl.
Blend the dressing ingredients well. Add to the salad, toss to combine and serve with crusty French bread.
1 090 kJ per serving

● High in fibre.

Suitable for: low gluten, low cholesterol (use kingklip instead of crayfish).

Pasta and rice

For substantial, filling dishes packed with fibre and vitamins, you cannot do better than use pasta and rice of all kinds.
There are different kinds of rice for different purposes: arborio for risottos and pilafs, for example, 'sticky' rice for rice pudding, or long-grained white rice for yellow rice with raisins. Wild rice, actually a grain, adds texture and interest to rice dishes.
Pasta may be white, brown or green (and every shade in between); with or without egg; freshly made or dried … the choice is yours.

Risotto with mushrooms
(Serves 4)

Make this risotto even more substantial by adding strips of roasted and skinned red sweet pepper, brinjals, baby marrows and tomatoes.

30 ml olive oil
1 small onion, peeled and chopped
1 clove garlic, crushed
400 g uncooked arborio or other risotto rice

50 ml dry white wine
5 ml fresh mixed herbs
20 g dried porcini mushrooms, soaked in 250 ml boiling water
1 litre chicken or vegetable stock
400 g button mushrooms, wiped and sliced
10 ml olive oil
fresh basil or rocket to garnish
Parmesan cheese and coarsely ground black pepper

Heat the oil in a large, heavy-based frying pan. Sauté the onion and garlic until softened but not browned. Add the rice and stir-fry for 1 minute. Add the wine and herbs, then the drained porcini mushrooms. Stir to combine. Add the hot stock, a spoonful at a time, and simmer while stirring. Keep on adding the stock to the rice until it has all been absorbed; this should take about 20 minutes.
Fry the fresh mushrooms in heated oil for 2 minutes and fold into the rice mixture. The rice should still be slightly moist and creamy. Turn into a warmed serving dish and decorate with basil leaves or rocket.
Serve with grated Parmesan cheese and coarsely ground black pepper.
900 kJ per serving

● The water in which the dried mushrooms were soaked may be used as part of the stock. No extra salt is needed, because stock is usually quite salty.
● The stock must be kept at boiling point while adding it to the rice.
● For a low-salt diet, use boiling water or low-salt chicken stock (recipe on page 149).
● High in fibre.

Suitable for: low gluten, low cholesterol, low fat.

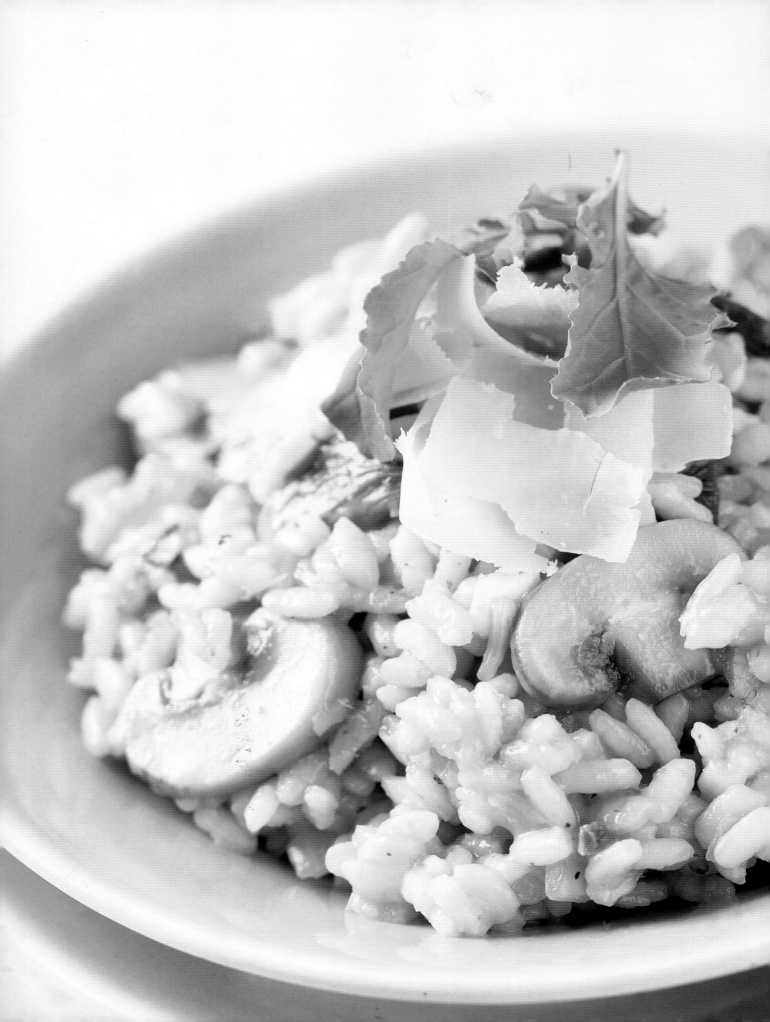

Pineapple and pecan rice salad with curry dressing

(Serves 4)

To add an even crunchier taste, use a mixture of brown and wild rice instead of brown rice only.

250 ml brown rice, cooked until tender
½ medium pineapple, peeled and chopped
4 spring onions, trimmed and chopped
1 small red or green apple, cored and chopped
250 ml chopped pecan nuts
30 ml chopped seedless raisins

DRESSING
65 ml oil
45 ml white vinegar
15 ml curry powder
10-20 ml sugar

Combine the rice and pineapple with the remaining ingredients in a large bowl. Mix in the dressing just before serving. To make the dressing, combine all the ingredients in a screw-top jar and shake well.
900 kJ per serving

● This dish is fibre-rich.

Suitable for: low gluten.

Brown rice pancakes

(Serves 4)

These unusual pancakes may be served on their own as an accompaniment, or with a sweet or savoury topping.

125 ml self-raising flour
125 ml cooked brown rice
2 eggs, lightly beaten
30 ml low-fat milk
60 ml butter or canola oil

Sift the flour and make a well in the centre. Combine the rice, eggs and milk and place in the well. Gradually incorporate the mixture into the flour, until well combined. Melt the butter or oil in a large frying pan. Drop heaped tablespoonfuls of rice mixture into the pan. Flatten them slightly and cook for 2 minutes on each side. Remove and keep warm while making the rest. Serve with roast meats or poultry, or cool and serve with sweet or savoury toppings.
400 kJ per pancake

● High in fibre.

Suitable for: low cholesterol, low fat.

Spaghetti with fresh tomato sauce

(Serves 4)

Spaghetti goes particularly well with tomato sauce – in this case, an excellent basic sauce that can be used in many other dishes.

400 g spaghetti or tagliatelle
125 ml grated Parmesan cheese

SAUCE
4 large ripe tomatoes
125 ml chopped pitted black olives
2 cloves garlic, crushed
60 ml shredded fresh basil
50 ml olive oil
pinch sugar
salt and pepper to taste

First make the tomato sauce. Pour boiling water over the tomatoes and leave for 1 minute. Drain, then plunge the tomatoes into cold water and pull off the skins. Squeeze out and discard the seeds and chop the flesh roughly. Mix with the remaining sauce ingredients and heat until just boiling. Cover and keep warm.
Cook the pasta until al dente. Drain and toss with the tomato sauce and serve with the Parmesan cheese.
650 kJ per serving

● For a low-sodium diet, omit the olives and salt in the sauce.

Suitable for: low fat, low cholesterol.

Pasta and roasted vegetables
(Serves 6)

A luscious combination of pasta and vegetables that will conjure up images of a Tuscan summer.

2 red onions, or other mild onions, peeled and cut into wedges
1 clove garlic
1 large red or yellow sweet pepper, cored, seeded and cut into strips
4 baby marrows, washed and sliced
2 large ripe tomatoes, quartered
4 small leeks, trimmed and sliced
100 g button mushrooms, wiped and sliced
5 ml mixed fresh herbs
salt and coarsely ground black pepper to taste
50 ml extra-virgin olive oil
400 g bow tie pasta
8 fresh basil leaves to garnish
shaved or grated Parmesan cheese

Preheat the oven to 200 °C.
Combine all the vegetables in an ovenproof baking pan. Sprinkle the herbs, salt and pepper over, then drizzle the oil over. Roast for 30 minutes.
Meanwhile, cook the pasta in plenty of salted boiling water until al dente (just done). Drain the pasta and place on a large serving platter. Top with the roasted vegetables, garnish with basil leaves and serve with shaved or grated Parmesan cheese.
800 kJ per serving

● High in fibre.

Suitable for: low fat, low cholesterol.

Pasta with ostrich bolognese sauce
(Serves 4)

Using lean ostrich mince instead of steak or topside mince brings this dish within the ambit of healthy eating even if one has to keep a check on fat intake.

1 onion, peeled and chopped
30 ml canola oil
500 g ostrich mince
fresh tomato sauce (see Spaghetti with fresh tomato sauce, page 127)
salt and freshly ground black pepper to taste
30 ml chopped parsley

Stir-fry the onion in heated oil until softened but not browned. Add the ostrich mince and fry until just done. Add the tomato sauce and heat through, seasoning if necessary and garnishing with chopped parsley. Serve over cooked pasta of your choice.
800 kJ per serving

Suitable for: low fat, low cholesterol.

● For a low-kilojoule diet, omit the olives and halve the quantity of olive oil. Use a nonstick pan.

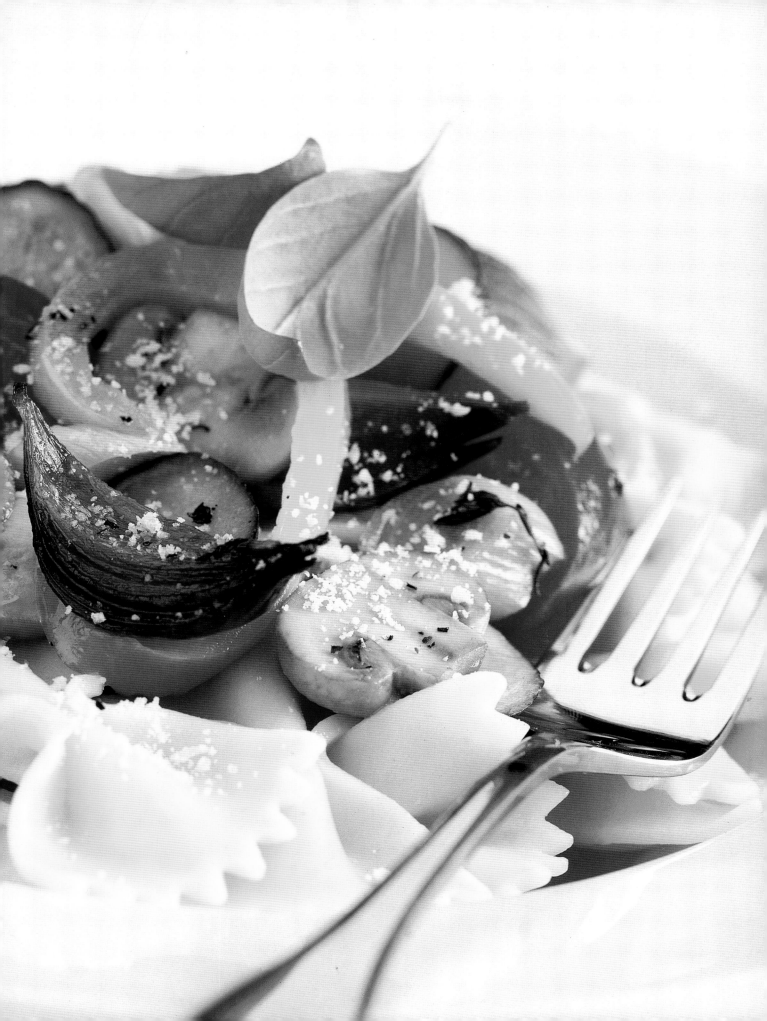

Penne with mushroom pepper sauce

(Serves 2)

The recipe may be doubled to serve four.

250 g penne rigate, cooked until al dente

SAUCE
15 ml olive oil
1 clove garlic, crushed
1 medium red sweet pepper, cored, seeded and sliced
1 medium green or orange sweet pepper, cored, seeded and sliced
750 g large black mushrooms, wiped and sliced
65 ml dry red wine
10 ml Worcestershire sauce
5 ml salt
freshly ground black pepper
15 ml chopped fresh parsley

First make the sauce. Heat the oil in a saucepan, add the garlic and peppers and cook until the peppers are just tender. Add the mushrooms and cook for 1 minute. Add the wine, Worcestershire sauce, seasoning and parsley, then cover and simmer over low heat for 5 minutes. Serve over hot penne.
750 kJ per serving

● This dish is fibre-rich.

Suitable for: low fat, low cholesterol.

Baking

Baked goodies smell and taste so marvellous that it seems they're almost guaranteed to be bad for you … While there's usually a lot of hidden saturated fats in cakes, biscuits, tarts and so on, there are ways to enjoy your favourite bakes without overstepping the boundaries. The recipes in this chapter offer some solutions.

Orange polenta and almond cake

(Serves 6)

This cake has an excellent flavour and texture.

220 g butter or margarine
220 g castor sugar
4 eggs
200 g finely ground almonds
5 ml vanilla essence
150 g polenta
grated peel and juice of ½ orange
5 ml gluten-free baking powder (recipe on page 149)

Preheat the oven to 180 °C.
Beat the butter or margarine and sugar until light and fluffy. Beat in the eggs, one at a time, then stir in the ground almonds and vanilla essence and mix well. Fold in the polenta, orange peel and juice and the baking powder.
Turn the batter into a lightly greased 20 cm diameter springform cake pan and bake for 60 minutes. Remove from the oven and cool in the pan for a few minutes, then turn out onto a wire rack and cool completely.
1 600 kJ per serving
Suitable for: low gluten.

Ricotta cheesecake

(Serves 12)

If you mourn the loss of cheesecake on your reduced-fat diet, this cake fills the gap admirably!

250 ml macaroons (recipe on page 134)
30 ml sugar
30 ml melted margarine

FILLING
375 ml ricotta cheese
250 ml low-fat natural yoghurt
4 egg whites
250 ml sugar
15 ml cornflour

5 ml vanilla essence
45 ml lemon juice

Preheat the oven to 180 °C.

Mix the macaroons, sugar and margarine well and press firmly into the base of a 25 cm diameter springform pan very lightly sprayed with nonstick cooking spray. Chill in the refrigerator.

Make the filling. Purée approximately ⅓ of the ricotta cheese, all the yoghurt and the egg whites until very smooth. Add the remaining ricotta a little at a time, blending until smooth after each addition. Gradually blend in the sugar and cornflour, then blend in the vanilla essence and lemon juice.

Pour the filling into the crust in the springform cake pan and bake for 80 minutes. The cake must feel firm near the centre when lightly touched.

Turn off the oven and leave the cake to cool in the oven, with the door ajar, for at least 2 hours. Transfer the cake to the refrigerator and release the sides of the pan once cold. Serve with fresh berries of your choice.

885 kJ per serving

● The cake will fall to approximately half its height after chilling.

Suitable for: low cholesterol, low gluten.

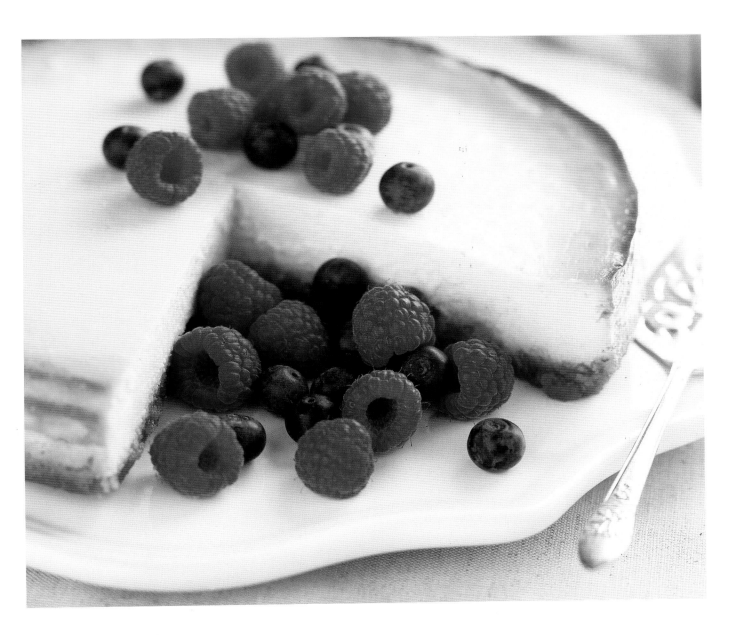

Angel cake

(Serves 8-10)

This cake is light as air and absolutely delicious.

120 g cake flour
250 g fine granulated sugar
10 egg whites
5 ml cream of tartar
2 ml salt
1 ml almond essence or 2 ml vanilla essence

Preheat the oven to 160 °C.
Sift the flour and half the sugar together several times to incorporate as much air as possible.
In a separate bowl, beat the egg whites until foamy, then add the cream of tartar and salt and continue beating until the egg whites are stiff but not dry.
Add 25 ml of the remaining sugar to the egg whites and beat well. Continue adding the sugar, 25 ml at a time and beating after each addition, until all the sugar has been incorporated.
Sift the flour and sugar mixture in thin layers over the egg whites and fold in each layer carefully.
Fold in the almond or vanilla essence.
Spoon the mixture carefully into an ungreased tube pan, 240 mm in diameter, and bake for 1 hour.
Invert the pan onto a cooling rack and cool the cake in the pan for approximately 1 hour. Loosen the cake carefully from the sides of the pan and remove the pan.
610 kJ per serving

Chocolate angel cake: Sift 80 ml sifted cocoa powder and 10 ml sifted instant coffee powder with the flour and half the sugar. Continue as described in the recipe.

● Tap the pan lightly on a flat surface before baking to remove any big air bubbles.

Suitable for: low cholesterol.

Whole-wheat date and raisin loaf

(Makes 2 loaves)

A delightfully crunchy new take on the old-fashioned date loaf.

300 ml boiling water
40 ml margarine or butter
5 ml bicarbonate of soda
450 g dates, stoned and finely chopped
3 eggs
250 ml brown sugar
750 g unsifted whole-wheat flour
10 ml baking powder
2 ml salt
10 ml vanilla essence
500 ml chopped pecan nuts or walnuts
65 ml seedless raisins

Preheat the oven to 180 °C.
Pour the water into a large mixing bowl and stir in the margarine or butter and bicarbonate of soda. Stir in the dates, eggs and brown sugar and mix well. Stir in the flour, baking powder and salt, then the vanilla essence, chopped nuts and raisins, blending thoroughly.
Pour the mixture into 2 large loaf pans, greased or sprayed with nonstick cooking spray. Bake on the middle shelf of the oven for 80 minutes.
Leave to cool slightly in the pans, then turn the loaves out onto a wire rack to cool completely.
To serve, slice and spread with butter.
860 kJ per serving

● High in fibre.

Suitable for: low cholesterol.

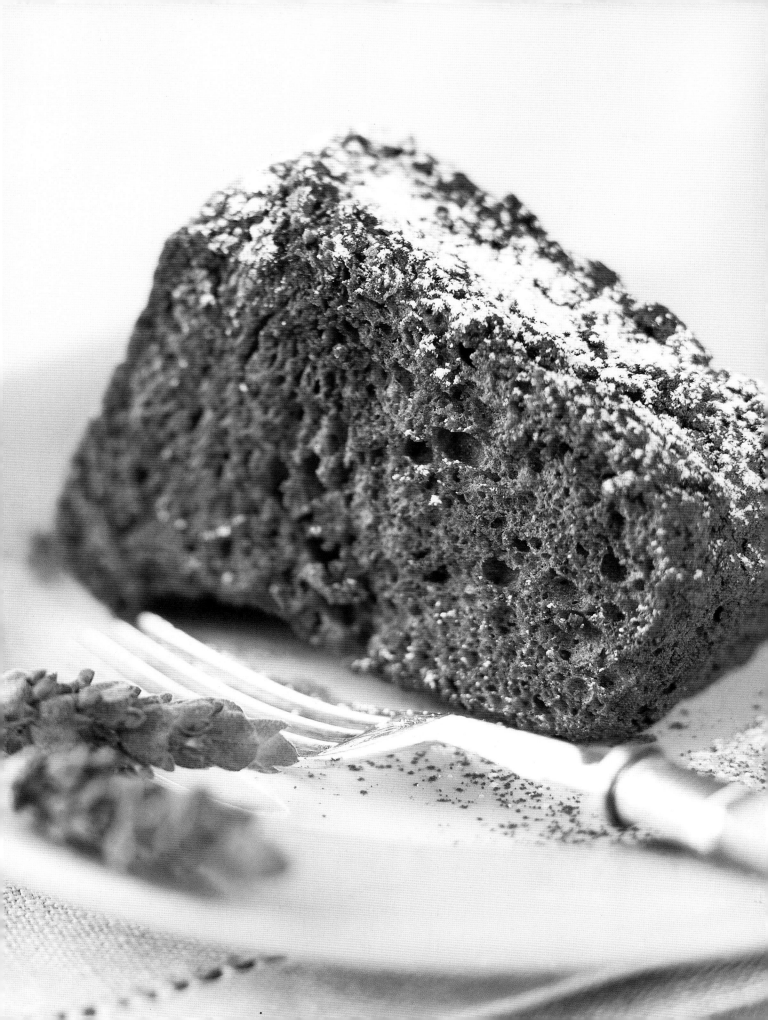

Almond macaroons

(Makes about 30)

Melting almond-flavoured mouthfuls of pure bliss!

250 g ground almonds
2 ml salt
250 g caster sugar
4 egg whites
5 ml almond essence

Preheat the oven to 150 °C.
Combine the almonds, salt and caster sugar in a sauce-pan. Heat over low heat until warm, then stir to mix well. Whisk the egg whites until foamy and slightly stiff, add to almond mixture and mix well. Stir in the almond essence.
Line a baking sheet with baking parchment. Spoon tea-spoonfuls of the egg white mixture onto the baking sheet and bake for 20 minutes. Remove from the oven, then use a spatula to transfer the macaroons from the paper to a cooling rack. Leave to cool.
450 kJ per serving

Suitable for: low gluten.

Muffins

(Makes 12)

These crunchy muffins are an excellent source of fibre and B vitamins.

200 ml whole-wheat flour
250 ml cake flour
25 ml baking powder
2 ml salt
125 ml low-fat milk
1 egg, well beaten
75 ml canola oil
65 ml honey

Preheat the oven to 200 °C.
Stir the whole-wheat flour, cake flour, baking powder and salt together in a mixing bowl.
Combine the milk, egg, oil and honey and add to the dry ingredients in the bowl. Stir until just moistened. Fill greased muffin pans to ⅔ full and bake for 20 minutes, or until golden brown and springy to the touch. Allow to cool for a few minutes, then remove from the pans. Serve on their own, or buttered.
280 kJ per serving

● These muffins are high in fibre.

VARIATIONS: ADD WASHED FRESH BLUEBERRIES, OR GRATED CARROT, OR BRAN AND SEEDLESS RAISINS TO THE DRY INGREDIENTS.

Suitable for: low cholesterol, diabetics.

Microwave oatmeal squares

(Makes 25 squares)

Quick, easy, crunchy – and good for you!

125 ml margarine
2 ml almond or vanilla essence
125 ml soft brown sugar
500 ml oats

Place the margarine in a 2 litre square microwave-safe dish and microwave on 100% power for 40-60 seconds, or until melted.
Stir in the almond or vanilla essence and sugar and mix well. Stir in the oats and mix well.
Press the mixture firmly into the prepared pan and micro-wave on 100% power for 5 minutes. Remove from micro-wave oven and allow to cool. Cut into squares.
300 kJ per serving

To bake in a conventional oven: Preheat the oven to 180 °C. Melt the margarine then mix with the almond or vanilla essence and sugar, and then the oats. Press into a pan and bake for 15 minutes, or until browned and bubbling.

● High in fibre.

Suitable for: low cholesterol.

Whole-wheat buttermilk rusks

(Makes about 50 rusks)

1 kg unsifted whole-wheat flour
250 g cake flour
10 ml baking powder
10 ml bicarbonate of soda
10 ml cream of tartar
10 ml salt
250 g margarine
125 ml seedless raisins
2 eggs
375 ml sugar
500 ml low-fat buttermilk
250 ml canola oil

Preheat the oven to 190 °C.
Combine all the dry ingredients, except the sugar, in a large mixing bowl.
Cut the margarine into small pieces and rub it into the dry ingredients until the mixture resembles fine breadcrumbs. Add the raisins.
Beat the eggs, sugar, buttermilk and oil together. Combine with the dry ingredients to form a stiff dough.
Shape into balls and pack close together in a greased loaf pan. Bake for 45 minutes. Turn out of the pan, allow to cool for 30 minutes and break into individual rusks. Dry out in the oven at 100 °C for 4-5 hours, or overnight in the warming drawer. Cool completely and store in airtight containers.
400 kJ per serving

- The sugar may be omitted, or the quantity decreased.
- These rusks are high in fibre.

Suitable for: low cholesterol.

Scones with oil

(Makes 12)

One is inclined to overmix scones – which results in heavy, stodgy scones. This recipe removes most of the temptation to overmix, and produces really light scones.

500 ml cake flour
20 ml baking powder
2 ml salt
100 ml canola oil
1 large egg
125 ml milk

Preheat the oven to 240 °C.
Sift the flour, baking powder and salt together.
Combine the oil, egg and milk in a bowl. Add to the dry ingredients and cut into the flour mixture, using a round-bladed knife or a pastry cutter. Do not knead. Mix lightly, then drop tablespoonfuls onto a greased baking sheet. Bake for 10 minutes.
300 kJ per serving

VARIATIONS
- TO MAKE WHOLE-WHEAT SCONES (HIGH IN FIBRE), USE 250 ML UNSIFTED WHOLE-WHEAT FLOUR AND 250 ML CAKE FLOUR INSTEAD OF CAKE FLOUR ONLY.
- TO MAKE CHEESE SCONES, ADD 125 ML GRATED REDUCED-FAT CHEDDAR CHEESE TO THE DRY INGREDIENTS.

Suitable for: low cholesterol.

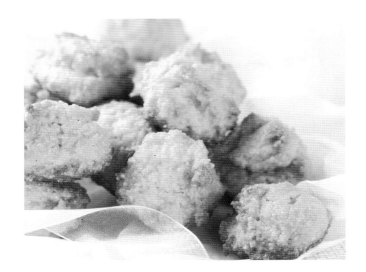

Whole-wheat tortillas

(Makes 12)

Tortillas are useful 'packages' for all kinds of fillings. Make a supply and freeze them, interleaved with waxed paper or plastic, until needed.

375 ml white bread flour
375 ml whole-wheat flour
250 ml water

Combine the white bread flour and whole-wheat flour in a bowl or on a board. Make a well in the centre, add the water and work it into the flour. Knead until smooth and pliable. Divide into 12 equal-sized balls and roll each out into rounds on a lightly floured board.

Heat an ungreased griddle or cast-iron frying pan. Cook the tortillas, one at a time, turning with a fish slice or spatula when the underside is golden, about 2 minutes, and cook on the other side. Remove the tortilla and keep warm between tea towels, or in a low oven, until ready to serve.
280 kJ per serving

- Interleave with plastic, overwrap and freeze for up to 1 month.
- High in fibre.

Suitable for: low cholesterol.

Rosemary breadsticks

(Makes 14)

Make the breadsticks in advance and store them for up to 2 weeks in an airtight container. They are great with soups and stews, and can also be served as an accompaniment to starters such as brinjal pâté (recipe on page 67).

500 g cake flour
5 g instant dried yeast (½ x 10 g packet)
300 ml warm water
30 ml olive or canola oil
1 egg, beaten with 30 ml water
45 ml very finely chopped fresh rosemary
coarse salt

In a large bowl, mix half the flour with yeast and add the water. Mix until smooth. Add the oil, 30 ml of the egg mixture (reserve the remainder for glazing) and the rosemary. Mix in enough of the remaining flour, 125 ml at a time, to make a soft dough. Knead on a lightly floured surface until smooth and elastic, about 8 minutes. Grease a large bowl with oil, place the dough in it and turn the dough around to coat the surface of the dough with oil. Allow to rise, covered, for 30 minutes. Preheat the oven to 200 °C.

Halve the dough. Roll each half out into a rope 40 cm long and cut it into 14 pieces. Roll each piece into a rope 30 cm long. Make each breadstick by twisting 2 ropes together. Place on a greased baking sheet. Repeat until all the breadsticks have been twisted. Brush with reserved egg mixture and sprinkle with coarse salt.

Bake for 15 minutes, or until the breadsticks are golden. Transfer to a wire rack to cool completely.
450 kJ per serving

VARIATIONS
- TRY DRIED HERBS SUCH AS THYME OR CORIANDER INSTEAD OF THE ROSEMARY.
- USE HALF CAKE FLOUR AND HALF WHOLE-WHEAT FLOUR.

Suitable for: low cholesterol, low fat.

Pancakes

(Makes about 25)

Pancakes are a marvellous stand-by, so why not make a batch or two and store them in your freezer, ready to use when needed?

500 ml cake flour
2 ml salt
2 ml baking powder
2 eggs
650 ml milk
30 ml melted butter or oil
15 ml brandy (optional)
oil for baking

Combine the cake flour, salt and baking powder in a bowl.

Beat the eggs and milk together in a separate bowl. Gradually add to the dry ingredients, beating all the time. Beat in the melted butter or oil and the brandy (if using). Leave the batter to stand for 1 hour before making the pancakes.

Preheat a heavy-based frying pan and grease lightly with oil. Pour a thin layer of the batter into the pan, tilting it to distribute the batter evenly.

Bake on one side until lightly browned, about 2 minutes, then turn the pancake over with a fish slice or spatula and bake for another minute.

Turn the pancake out onto a plate and keep warm over a saucepan of boiling water or, covered, in the oven at 100 °C. Continue until all the batter has been used.

Serve with cinnamon sugar, or with a sweet or savoury filling of your choice.
280 kJ per serving

- The pan only needs greasing once.
- Freeze pancakes interleaved with waxed paper or plastic. Overwrap securely in foil or plastic.
- To serve after freezing, remove the wrapping and interleaving sheets. Heat for 30 seconds on either side in a warm frying pan, or in the oven at 100 °C or on a plate over boiling water for at least 30 minutes. You can also reheat pancakes, a few at a time, in the microwave on 100% power for a couple of seconds.

Low-cholesterol waffles
(Makes 8)

Using a nonstick waffle iron and egg whites only, instead of whites and yolks, helps these waffles to score low down on the fats scale.

3 egg whites
500 ml low-fat buttermilk
120 g cake flour
120 g whole-wheat flour
10 ml baking powder
5 ml bicarbonate of soda
65 ml oil

Heat a nonstick waffle iron. Whisk the egg whites until frothy and fold in the remaining ingredients until smooth.

Pour 125 ml batter onto the centre of the waffle iron and make sure that the batter is evenly distributed. Close the waffle iron and bake the waffle for about 5 minutes. Remove the waffle and keep warm while making the remaining waffles.
800 kJ per serving

Suitable for: low cholesterol.

Mexican mealie meal bread
(Serves 12)

In Mexico, cornmeal would be used to make this loaf. Yellow mealie meal makes an excellent alternative.

750 ml yellow unsifted mealie meal
30 ml sugar
30 ml baking powder
20 ml salt
6 eggs
350 ml canola oil
500 ml low-fat natural yoghurt
250 g canned cream-style sweetcorn
250 ml finely chopped onion
250 ml finely chopped red sweet pepper
250 ml (1 cup) grated low-fat cheese

Preheat the oven to 180 °C.

Combine all the dry ingredients in a large mixing bowl. Beat the eggs, oil and yoghurt in another bowl, and stir in the sweetcorn. Stir the dry ingredients into the egg mixture. Mix well, then add the onion and red pepper. Turn half the batter into a greased pie dish or cake pan and sprinkle the grated cheese over. Spread the rest of the batter over the cheese. Bake for 1 hour. Cool briefly in the pan, then turn out onto a wire rack and cool completely.
450 kJ per serving

- Yellow mealie meal may be difficult to find. Try health shops, or use polenta, which is available at many supermarkets.

Mealie meal muffins: Spoon the batter into muffin pans, to fill them to ⅔ full, and bake for 30 minutes.

Suitable for: low gluten.

Steamed maize bread

(Serves 8)

This loaf was traditionally steamed in old-fashioned metal cocoa tins, with a lid. In the absence of these tins, a loaf pan or casserole dish, tightly covered, may be used instead.

750 ml minced fresh mealie kernels
5 ml salt
15 ml sugar
7 ml gluten-free baking powder
15 ml melted butter or margarine
1 beaten egg

Combine the mealies, salt, sugar and baking powder. Stir in the melted butter or margarine and egg. Mix well. Grease a loaf pan and spoon in the mixture. Cover well with two layers of thick aluminium foil and tie securely with string. Place the loaf pan in a large saucepan and add enough boiling water to come halfway up the sides of the loaf pan. Cover with the lid and steam the bread for 1½-2 hours. Remove from the saucepan, allow to cool slightly then remove the foil and turn the loaf out. Slice, butter and serve.
420 kJ per serving

Suitable for: low gluten, low fat.

Desserts

To most of us, desserts are the high point of any meal. This becomes a problem when we have to count kilojoules or watch fat and cholesterol levels … and, usually, simply served fresh fruit is the panacea for all ills. But fresh fruit ad nauseum can be boring, even if it has the health bonus of usually being high in fibre, so here are some more interesting (but still healthy) hot and cold desserts to tempt your palate.

COLD DESSERTS

The selection ranges from snows and roulades to tempting 'creams' and ices, but you can rest assured that none of the dishes is high in fats or kilojoules.

Tropical fruit brûlée

(Serves 4)

It tastes so divine that you'll forget there's no cream in this 'brûlée'!

3 kiwi fruit, peeled and sliced
12 litchis, peeled, stoned and halved
2 ripe bananas, peeled and sliced
40 ml unsweetened granadilla or peach juice
400 ml low-fat Greek-style yoghurt
1 small ripe papino or mango, peeled and seeded
  or stoned, then cut into chunks
½ pineapple, peeled and cut into chunks
100 ml soft brown sugar for sprinkling

Layer the kiwi fruit, litchis and bananas in 4 sundae glasses or glass dishes. Drizzle a little granadilla or peach juice over each, and top with 50 ml yoghurt.
Layer the papino or mango and pineapple on top. Drizzle the remaining granadilla or peach juice over, spread the remaining yoghurt on top, then sprinkle thickly with soft brown sugar (25 ml to each dessert).
Refrigerate at least 12 hours, to give the sugar time to form a 'brûlée' crust on top.
765 kJ per serving

● High in fibre.

VARIATIONS
● RICOTTA CHEESE MAY BE USED INSTEAD OF THE YOGHURT.
● A LITTLE COINTREAU OR BRAMBLE LIQUEUR MAY BE USED INSTEAD OF GRANADILLA OR PEACH JUICE.

Fruit and muesli sundae: Reduce the quantity of yoghurt to 160 ml (40 ml for each dessert) and layer 40 ml (10 ml each) muesli (recipe on page 148) over each yoghurt layer in the dessert. Omit the sugar.

Suitable for: low cholesterol (use low-fat yoghurt), low gluten.

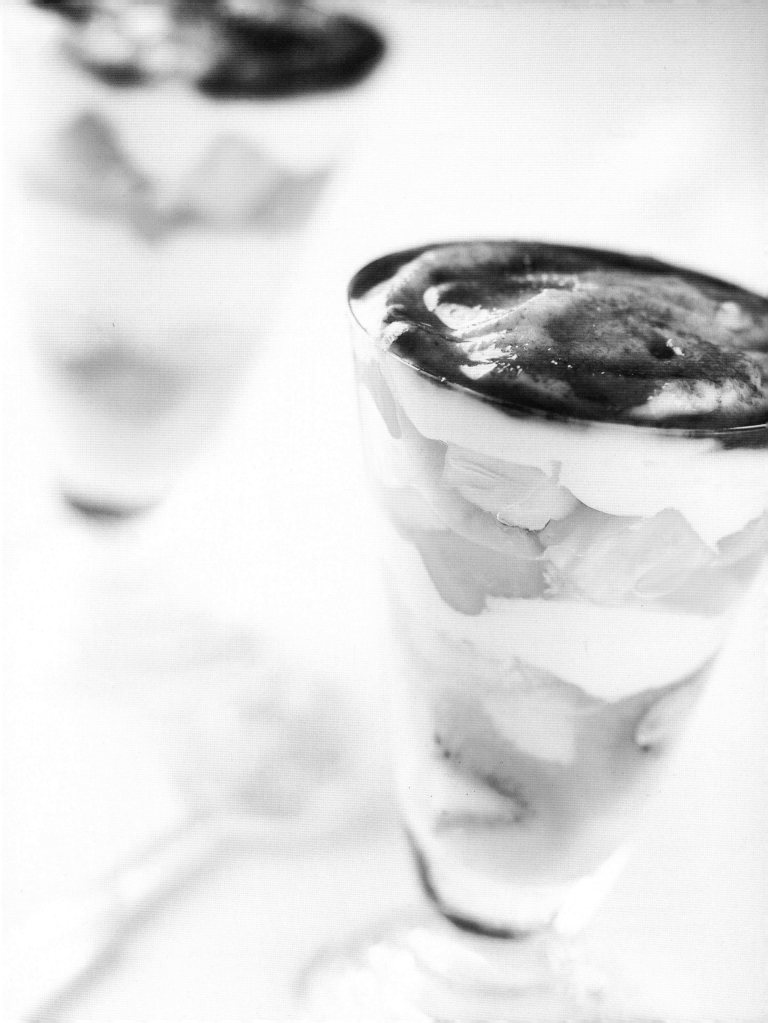

Berry jellies

(Serves 4)

Although any fruit may be used, berries add a richness of flavour, aroma and colour that's hard to beat.

250 ml fresh boysenberries, raspberries or youngberries, washed well
200 ml unsweetened berry or peach juice
1 x 80 g packet port wine, blackcurrant or other dark red jelly powder
boiling water

Rinse the berries in cold water and drain in a colander or sieve. Place in a dish – preferably in a single layer – and pour the fruit juice over. Macerate for at least 6 hours.
Make up the jelly, using 225 ml boiling water. Drain the berries carefully and add the fruit juice to the jelly. Stir to mix well.
Divide the berries between 4 individual dishes and pour the jelly over. Place in the refrigerator until starting to set, then stir carefully to distribute the berries more evenly in the jelly. Return to the refrigerator and leave until set.
Remove from the refrigerator 15 minutes before serving. Serve low-fat natural yoghurt and ricotta cheese separately.
270 kJ per serving

Suitable for: low cholesterol, low fat, low gluten.

Strawberry pavlovas

(Serves 4-6)

If you wish, add a little liqueur of your choice to the fruit.

3 egg whites
175 g caster sugar
5 ml cornflour
1 ml vanilla essence

FILLING
1 kiwi fruit, peeled and sliced
275 g strawberries, hulled and sliced
100 g raspberries or youngberries
30 ml orange juice
150 ml low-fat Greek-style yoghurt

Preheat the oven to 140 °C.
Line a baking sheet with nonstick baking parchment or greased foil, shiny side under. Draw 4-6 rounds on the paper. Whisk the egg whites until soft peaks form. Gradually whisk in two-thirds of the sugar, until glossy. Sprinkle the cornflour over and fold in gently with the vanilla essence and remaining sugar.
Spread mounds of egg white mixture over each round. Using a spoon, gently scoop a hollow in the centre of each. Bake for 45 minutes, or until just golden. Cool completely on the baking sheet before removing.
Mix the kiwi fruit and strawberries with the raspberries and orange juice. Spoon the yoghurt into the meringue nests and arrange the fruit on top. Serve immediately.
800 kJ per serving

VARIATION: ANY COMBINATION OF FRUITS MAY BE USED.

Suitable for: low fat, low cholesterol (use fat-free yoghurt), low gluten.

Lemon snow

(Serves 4)

15 ml gelatine powder
65 ml cold water
250 ml hot water
250 ml sugar
65 ml lemon juice
grated peel of ½ lemon
2 egg whites, stiffly whisked

Soak the gelatine in the cold water until spongy, then dissolve it in the hot water. Stir in the sugar, lemon juice and grated lemon peel and strain through a fine sieve into a bowl. Chill in the refrigerator until starting to set, then beat until light and foamy, using an egg whisk. Fold the egg whites into the mixture and pour into a dampened mould or individual moulds. Chill until set. Serve with a thin custard.
580 kJ per serving

VARIATION: USE ORANGE JUICE AND PEEL INSTEAD OF LEMON.

Suitable for: low cholesterol.

Plum snow

(Serves 4)

If you prefer a less tart result, use late yellow plums or greengages instead of red plums.

500 ml plum purée
2 jumbo egg whites
10 ml cinnamon sugar

Place the plum purée in a large bowl.
Whisk the egg whites with the cinnamon sugar until very stiff.
Fold the egg whites carefully into the plum purée and transfer to 4 individual glasses or glass dishes.
Chill in the refrigerator for at least 1 hour before serving.
700 kJ per serving

- Depending on their size, you will need 4-8 plums to make 500 ml purée. Wash the plums well, stone and chop them coarsely and place in a saucepan with 30-45 ml sugar. Bring to boil, then simmer until softened, 5-6 minutes. Purée the plums, including the skins.
- To make cinnamon sugar, mix 10-15 ml ground cinnamon with 60 ml white or brown sugar.
- Retaining the plum skin not only adds colour and fibre, but also provides antioxidant vitamin A.

Suitable for: low cholesterol, low gluten.

Fresh peaches with raspberry yoghurt sauce

(Serves 4)

The juxtaposition of sweet and tart in this simple dessert is absolutely divine.

4 ripe dessert peaches, peeled
fresh raspberries or mint to decorate
SAUCE
250 ml frozen, unsweetened raspberries
125 ml low-fat natural yoghurt
15 ml honey or brown sugar

First make the sauce. Purée the raspberries, yoghurt and honey or brown sugar until smooth. Refrigerate until needed.
Slice the peaches and place in 4 individual dishes. When ready to serve, spoon the sauce over or, alternatively, spread the sauce on plates and arrange the peaches on top. Decorate with fresh raspberries or mint and serve.
590 kJ per serving

- To make it easier to peel the peaches, first blanch them in boiling water.
- High in fibre.

Suitable for: low gluten, low cholesterol, low fat.

Grapefruit granita

(Serves 4-6)

Water ices tend to be tart rather than sweet, which is why they make such excellent palate fresheners after a meal. Lemons or oranges may be used instead of grapefruit.

white of 1 large egg
250 ml fresh grapefruit
20 ml freshly grated lemon peel
375 ml sugar
125 ml dry white wine
375 ml cold water

Whisk the egg white until frothy.
Combine all the ingredients in a large bowl and stir until the sugar has dissolved. Transfer to a freezer container and freeze until slushy. Beat well to remove ice crystals, then return to the container and freeze until firm.
Serve scoops of granita heaped in glass bowls, accompanied by wafers or paper-thin ginger biscuits.
675 kJ per serving

Suitable for: low cholesterol, low fat, low gluten, low sodium.

Apple cinnamon sorbet with strawberry coulis
(Serves 8)

A sweeter apple changes the flavour from tangy to mellow.

**250 ml peeled, cored and finely grated Golden
   Delicious apple
30 ml lemon juice
30 ml Calvados (optional)
2 ml ground cinnamon
625 ml water
250 ml granulated sugar
625 ml apple juice**

**COULIS
250 g fresh strawberries
icing sugar to taste (optional)**

Combine the apple, lemon juice, Calvados (if using) and cinnamon in a saucepan. Cook over moderate heat, stirring, until the apple is tender, about 3 minutes.
Bring the water and sugar to the boil in another saucepan and cook until the sugar has dissolved, stirring from time to time. Remove from the stove.
Stir in the apple mixture and apple juice. Freeze in a metal pan or bowl until barely firm. Beat by hand, or use an electric mixer, until slushy. Return to the freezer and freeze until firm.
Remove from the freezer 10 minutes before serving, to allow to soften slightly. Spoon into small dishes or glasses and drizzle the strawberry coulis over. Serve with sliced fresh fruit such as grapes or kiwi fruit.
To make the coulis, purée the strawberries until smooth, adding a little icing sugar if desired.
660 kJ per serving

Suitable for: low fat, low gluten.

Kiwi fruit water ice
(Serves 4-6)

Strawberries or fresh granadilla pulp make excellent alternatives to the kiwi fruit.

**8 medium kiwi fruit
250 ml sugar
250 ml water
250 ml dry white wine
250 ml water, extra**

Purée the kiwi fruit until smooth. Push the pulp through a sieve to remove the seeds, if desired. Place the sugar and water in a saucepan and stir over low heat, without boiling, until the sugar has dissolved. Bring to the boil, then boil rapidly for 3 minutes, without stirring. Remove the sugar syrup from the stove and cool for 5 minutes. Stir in the kiwi fruit pulp and the remaining ingredients. Pour into a freezer-proof container, cover with foil and freeze until the mixture is starting to set around the edges. Remove from the freezer, mix well with a fork, cover and freeze until firm.
Serve scoops in dessert glasses.
675 kJ per serving

Suitable for: low gluten, low sodium, low cholesterol, low fat.

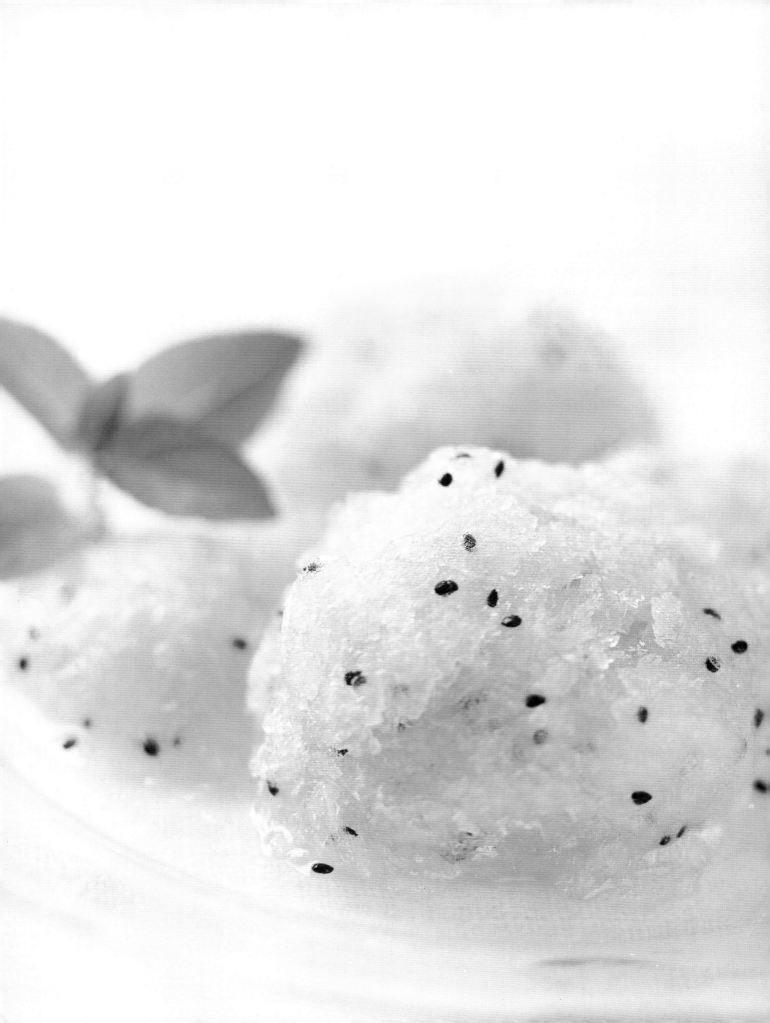

Pears baked in wine
(Serves 6)

Pears in red wine may also be served hot, with custard.

6 firm, ripe pears, peeled, cored and halved
**   lengthways**
10 ml lemon juice
125 ml dry red wine
250 ml clear honey
1 piece stick cinnamon
grated peel of ½ lemon

Preheat the oven to 190 °C.
Place the pears, cut side down, in a large shallow baking dish and sprinkle with the lemon juice.
Combine the wine, honey, cinnamon and grated lemon peel in a saucepan over moderate heat and bring to the boil, stirring now and then.
Pour the boiling syrup over the pears and cover the dish. Bake, basting occasionally, until the pears are tender when pricked with a sharp knife, about 20 minutes.
Cool the pears at room temperature, then chill in the refrigerator for 30 minutes. Remove the cinnamon stick before serving.
580 kJ per serving

● High in fibre.

Suitable for: low cholesterol.

Chocolate whip
(Serves 4)

A delightfully light, mousse-like dessert.

110 g plain or dark chocolate
25 ml milk
2 egg whites

Place the chocolate and milk in a saucepan and heat over low heat until the chocolate has melted, stirring once or twice. Remove from the stove and allow to cool. Whisk the egg whites until stiff, then fold them into the chocolate mixture. Pour into a serving bowl and chill

until set. Serve with whipped cream or low-fat natural yoghurt.
1 000 kJ per serving

VARIATION: USE ORANGE JUICE INSTEAD OF THE MILK.

Suitable for: low gluten.

Gooseberry fool
(Serves 4)

It's quick and easy to make and, best of all, it won't break the kilojoule bank.

500 ml low-fat natural yoghurt
15 ml caster sugar
25 ml rum or brandy (optional)
250 ml canned gooseberries, drained or fresh
**   gooseberries**
sprinkling of ground nutmeg

Whip the yoghurt, caster sugar and rum or brandy together until thick and smooth. Fold in the gooseberries and spoon the mixture into 4 serving dishes. Chill for 30 minutes. Sprinkle with a little nutmeg and serve.
700 kJ per serving

VARIATIONS
● ANY FRESH FRUIT MAY BE USED IN PLACE OF THE GOOSEBERRIES, E.G. 250 ML FINELY MASHED BANANAS, OR FRESH GRANADILLA PULP.
● KIRSCH, CALVADOS OR VAN DER HUM ARE EXCELLENT SUBSTITUTES FOR THE RUM OR BRANDY.

Suitable for: low cholesterol, low fat, low gluten.

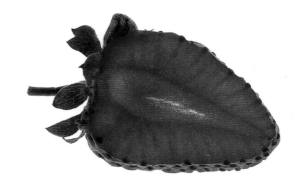

Peach mousse

(Serves 6)

Chilled mousses are a marvellous way to enjoy fruit on a balmy summer's evening. Nectarines, apricots, berries or plums may be used instead of peaches.

6 ripe peaches, peeled and stoned
½ x 80 g packet of lemon- or apricot-flavoured jelly
150 ml thick cream

Set 2 of the peaches aside and purée the remaining peaches. Make up the jelly with 145 ml boiling water and chill in the refrigerator until thick, but not completely set. Beat the jelly well with a rotary beater.
In a separate bowl, whip the cream until firm enough to hold its shape. Whisk into the jelly, then fold in the peach purée. Transfer to a serving bowl and leave to set. Just before serving, slice the 2 whole peaches and arrange them on top of the mousse.
910 kJ per serving

Suitable for: low sodium.

Chocolate cream

(Serves 6)

A light, low-fat creamy dessert that goes well with fresh berries.

45 ml cornflour
20 ml cocoa powder
500 ml low-fat milk
125 ml sugar
5 ml vanilla essence

Combine the cornflour and cocoa powder in a bowl. Whisk in the milk. Heat over moderate heat, stirring all the time, until smooth and thick. Stir in the sugar and vanilla essence and pour into small coffee cups. Chill well before serving.
480 kJ per serving

Suitable for: low cholesterol, low gluten.

Mango meringue roulade

(Serves 6)

It looks spectacular, but is really easy to make and tastes divine.

3 large egg whites
175 g caster sugar
5 ml cornflour
5 ml balsamic vinegar
5 ml vanilla extract
icing sugar to dust

FILLING
200 ml low-fat natural yoghurt
1 large ripe mango, peeled, stoned and diced
4 granadillas, halved and pulp removed
raspberry sauce (recipe on page 141) to serve

Preheat the oven to 150 °C.
Line a 33 x 23 cm Swiss roll pan with nonstick baking parchment. Whisk the egg whites until frothy and doubled in volume, then gradually whisk in the caster sugar until the mixture is thick and shiny. Mix the cornflour, vinegar and vanilla extract and whisk into the egg whites.
Spoon the mixture into the pan and level the surface carefully, to avoid pushing out the air. Bake for 30 minutes, or until the surface is just firm. Remove from the oven, cover with damp greaseproof paper and leave for 10 minutes. Dust another sheet of greaseproof paper with icing sugar. Discard the damp paper and turn the meringue out onto the sugar-coated paper. Peel off the lining paper.
Spread the yoghurt over the meringue and scatter the mango pieces over. Drizzle the granadilla pulp over. Using the paper as a guide, roll up the roulade from one short end, keeping the join underneath.
Serve with raspberry sauce.
965 kJ per serving

VARIATION: USE FRESH DESSERT PEACHES OR NECTARINES INSTEAD OF MANGO.

Suitable for: low cholesterol, low fat.

HOT DESSERTS

Did you think that all those comforting hot puddings were a thing of the past? Not so, as our selection of recipes with health in mind will show.

Hot lemon soufflé
(Serves 4)

Soufflés wait for no one … but this one is so delicious that you'll want to eat it immediately anyway, which means that it won't have time to collapse.

75 ml hot milk
40 g sugar
15 ml cake flour
25 ml butter or margarine
pinch salt
2 egg yolks
grated peel and juice of 1 large lemon
20 ml finely chopped candied orange or lemon
   peel
2 egg whites, whisked until stiff

Preheat the oven to 180 °C.
Mix the hot milk and the sugar in a bowl until the sugar dissolves. Place the flour in a small saucepan and add the milk, stirring with a wooden spoon until smooth. Add the butter or margarine and heat gently, stirring constantly, until the sauce is thick and smooth. Add the salt, stir well and remove from the stove.
Beat in the egg yolks, one at a time, and pour in 50 ml lemon juice in a thin, steady stream at the same time, to prevent curdling. Stir in the lemon peel and the candied orange or lemon peel. Fold in the egg whites and pour into a well-greased soufflé dish.
Bake for 30 minutes, or until well risen and golden. Serve immediately.
200 kJ per serving

- Have the soufflé dish ready before starting to make the soufflé.
- The egg whites should be stiff and shiny, but not dry.

Apple crumble
(Serves 6)

This all-time favourite is just as delectable made with fresh berries of your choice.

1 kg canned unsweetened pie apples
grated peel of 1 lemon
125 ml seedless raisins, soaked in water for
   30 minutes
25 ml brown sugar
5 ml ground cinnamon

TOPPING
60 ml butter or margarine
110 g sugar
100 g rolled oats

Preheat the oven to 180 °C.
Combine the apples, lemon peel, raisins, sugar and ground cinnamon in a bowl, then transfer the mixture to a lightly greased pie dish.
To make the topping, first cream the butter or margarine and sugar in a bowl. Work in the oats with your fingertips to make a crumbly mixture. Sprinkle over the apple mixture.
Bake until heated through and the topping is lightly browned, about 45 minutes. Serve hot or cold, with cream or custard.
1 100 kJ per serving

- High in fibre.

Suitable for: low cholesterol (use margarine).

Fruit-stuffed apples
(Serves 6)

A slightly different version of the classic baked apple, which goes down particularly well on a chilly autumn evening.

6 large cooking or dessert apples, cored

STUFFING
100 g dried apricots, chopped and soaked
   overnight in 25 ml brandy or orange juice
20 ml soft brown sugar

15 ml sultanas
200 ml sweet wine or water

Preheat the oven to 180 °C.
Make a shallow cut around the circumference of each apple to prevent bursting during cooking.
To make the stuffing, mix the apricots and soaking liquid with the brown sugar and sultanas. Use to stuff the centre of the apples. Place in an ovenproof dish.
Pour the wine or water over, cover lightly and bake until the apples are tender, about 45 minutes. Baste from time to time with the cooking liquid.
Pour a little wine syrup over each serving and serve hot, with cream or low-fat natural yoghurt.
675 kJ per serving

● High in fibre.

Suitable for: low gluten, low cholesterol, low fat.

Lime pudding
(Serves 6)

30 ml butter or margarine
125 ml caster sugar
2 eggs, separated
30 ml self-raising flour
65 ml lime juice
65 ml water
200 ml low-fat milk

Preheat the oven to 160 °C.
Cream the butter or margarine, sugar and egg yolks in a small bowl until light and creamy. Stir in the sifted flour, lime juice, water and milk. Whisk the egg whites until soft peaks form, and fold gently into the mixture.
Pour into 6 lightly greased 125 ml capacity ovenproof dishes and bake for 35 minutes. Serve hot with low-fat custard or low-fat natural yoghurt.
880 kJ per serving

VARIATION: USE LEMON OR ORANGE JUICE INSTEAD OF LIME JUICE.

Apricot and almond pudding
(Serves 6)

A warmly comforting pud, just like mom used to make.

410 g can apricots in fruit juice
3 large eggs
40 g caster sugar
50 g cake flour
pinch of salt
425 ml skimmed milk
10 g skimmed milk powder
2 ml almond extract
15 ml almond liqueur (optional)
10 g flaked almonds
icing sugar for dusting

Preheat the oven to 190 °C, with the baking sheet placed on a high shelf.
Drain the apricot halves well and pat dry. Arrange, cut side down, in the base of a 20 cm square baking dish.
Whisk the eggs and sugar together until pale, frothy and doubled in volume. Sift the flour and a pinch of salt over and continue whisking until smooth. Add the milk, milk powder, almond extract and almond liqueur (if using) and whisk for 1-2 minutes. Pour the batter over the apricots and sprinkle the flaked almonds over. Place the dish on the preheated baking sheet and bake for 30-35 minutes, or until golden, puffed up and firm to the touch.
Allow to cool for about 20 minutes, then dust lightly with icing sugar and serve with low-fat natural yoghurt or low-fat custard.
775 kJ per serving

● High in fibre, especially if fresh fruit is used.

VARIATIONS
● USE FRESH APRICOTS INSTEAD OF CANNED.
● FRESH PEACHES OR NECTARINES MAY BE USED INSTEAD OF APRICOTS.

Suitable for: low fat.

Nectarines with meringue topping

(Serves 4)

Ripe peaches, apricots or figs would go equally well in this dessert.

4 ripe nectarines
500 ml unsweetened peach juice
1 piece stick cinnamon
2 cloves

MERINGUE TOPPING
3 egg whites, at room temperature
pinch salt
pinch cream of tartar
125 ml sugar

Halve, skin and stone the nectarines and poach in the peach juice with cinnamon and cloves until tender, about 15 minutes. Remove the cinnamon and cloves and transfer the nectarines and juice to an ovenproof dish.
To make the topping, whisk the egg whites with the remaining topping ingredients until stiff peaks form. Preheat the grill.
Spoon the meringue mixture over the nectarines and brown under the grill. Serve immediately.
950 kJ per serving

● High in fibre.

Suitable for: low cholesterol, low fat, low gluten.

Rhubarb with apples and strawberries

(Serves 8)

Rhubarb is a much-neglected ingredient, possibly because it is too tart for most tastes. Add apples and strawberries, however, and the result is much mellower.

grated peel and juice of 1 orange
500 g fresh rhubarb, trimmed and cut into 2,5 cm
**   lengths**
1 large Granny Smith or Golden Delicious apple,
**   peeled, cored and thinly sliced**

250 ml water
50 ml sugar
500 ml fresh strawberries, washed and hulled
125 ml low-fat natural yoghurt
25 ml soft brown sugar

Combine the orange peel and juice, rhubarb, apple, water and sugar in a saucepan. Cover and bring to the boil. Reduce the heat and simmer for 10 minutes, or until the fruit is tender, stirring occasionally. Remove from the stove and stir in the strawberries. Add more sugar to taste, if necessary.
Serve warm or at room temperature, topped with yoghurt and sprinkled with brown sugar.
700 kJ per serving

● High in fibre.

VARIATION: IF YOU CAN AFFORD TO SPLURGE OCCASIONALLY, SERVE WITH MASCARPONE OR CRÈME FRAÎCHE INSTEAD OF YOGHURT.

Suitable for: low cholesterol, low fat, low gluten.

Basics

The recipes contained in this chapter will prove useful, not only to promote a healthy lifestyle but also for those on special diets.

Health muesli

(Makes 750 g)

The original health breakfast, which is ideal served with low-fat natural yoghurt or buttermilk and a drizzle of honey.

125 ml dried apples
125 ml dried apricots
500 ml rolled oats
250 ml wheat flakes
30 ml wheat germ
65 ml digestive bran

125 ml seedless raisins or sultanas
125 ml chopped mixed nuts
125 ml skimmed milk powder

Chop the dried apples and apricots finely. Combine with remaining ingredients and store in an airtight container. 630 kJ per serving

VARIATION: ADD 30 ML FINELY CHOPPED MIXED NUTS TO THE MIXTURE.

Low-salt chicken stock
(Makes 1,5 litres)

If you are on a low-sodium diet, this stock will allow you to expand your repertoire of menus considerably.

2 kg chicken or turkey carcass and necks
3 litres cold water
bouquet garni (parsley, thyme and bay leaf)
1 clove garlic, crushed
2 cloves
6 peppercorns
2 leeks, trimmed and sliced
4 carrots, peeled and sliced
1 onion, peeled and sliced
3 stalks soup celery, trimmed and finely chopped
1 turnip, peeled and chopped

Place the chicken or turkey in a large saucepan. Add the water, spices and herbs. Bring slowly to the boil, then reduce the heat and simmer, covered, for 1 hour, skimming the scum from the surface when necessary. Add the vegetables and continue simmering for 1-1½ hours. Skim the scum from the surface and strain the stock through a fine sieve. Chill the stock until any fat on the surface solidifies. Remove the fat. Pack the stock into smaller containers and freeze until needed.

Suitable for: low-sodium, low fat.

Gluten-free baking powder

Indispensable for gluten-free diets.

85 g cornflour
85 g bicarbonate of soda
75 g cream of tartar
75 g tartaric acid

Mix all the ingredients together, then sieve them 2-3 times. Store in an airtight container, in a cool, dry place.

Mozzarella cheese sauce
(Makes about 375 ml)

This is an excellent lower-fat alternative to cheese sauce made with Cheddar cheese. Other reduced-fat cheeses may be used instead of mozzarella.

25 ml spreading margarine
30 ml all-purpose flour
250 ml skimmed milk
250 ml shredded low-fat mozzarella cheese
cayenne pepper

Melt the margarine in a saucepan over medium-low heat. Stir in the flour and mix well, then cook for 1 minute, stirring. Stir in the milk and cook over moderate heat, stirring, for 3-5 minutes, or until the mixture comes to a low boil and has thickened. Remove from the stove and stir in the cheese until melted. Season with cayenne pepper to taste.

VARIATION: FOR EXTRA BITE, ADD A KNIFE-TIP OF PREPARED MUSTARD (YOUR CHOICE OF STRENGTH).

Suitable for: low fat.

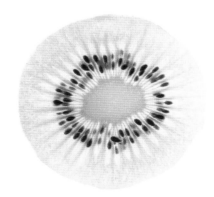

Home-made egg substitute
(65 ml = 1 whole egg)

6 egg whites
65 ml powdered fat-free milk
15 ml oil

Combine all the ingredients in a mixing bowl and blend until smooth. Store in a closed container in the refrigerator for up to 1 week, or freeze for up to 3 months.

Home-made tomato sauce (ketchup)
(Makes about 250 ml)

This recipe is low in sodium.

155 ml canned tomato paste
50 ml soft brown sugar
50 ml water
25 ml cider vinegar
1 ml mustard powder
1 ml ground cinnamon
pinch each ground allspice and ground cloves

Combine all the ingredients in a bowl or jar. Cover and store in the refrigerator for up to 1 month.

Yoghurt hollandaise
(Makes 300 ml)

A lower-fat alternative to Hollandaise sauce.

250 ml low-fat natural yoghurt
10 ml lemon juice
3 egg yolks
2 ml salt
2 ml Dijon mustard
pinch freshly ground pepper
15 ml chopped fresh parsley or dill

Beat the yoghurt, lemon juice and egg yolks in the top of a nonaluminium double boiler or in a heatproof glass bowl just big enough to fit in a small saucepan. Heat over sim-

mering water, stirring often, until the sauce has thickened, about 15 minutes. Remove from the stove and stir in the salt, mustard, pepper and parsley or dill. Serve warm.

● The sauce may be prepared in advance, refrigerated for up to 1 week, then reheated over hot, not simmering, water.

Light white sauce
(Makes 300 ml)

This white sauce contains almost no fat, and is useful to moisten all kinds of foods, from chicken to vegetables, and even desserts. It takes only a few minutes to make, and doesn't go lumpy.

25 ml cornflour or arrowroot
300 ml low-fat milk
2 ml salt

Place the cornflour or arrowroot in a saucepan. Add a little of the milk and stir until smooth. Add the remaining milk gradually, stirring to incorporate it completely. Bring to the boil, stirring continuously, then reduce the heat and simmer for 1 minute. Season with salt. Use while hot.

VARIATIONS
● ADD 30-45 ML FINELY CHOPPED CHIVES, DILL OR PARSLEY.
● ADD 10 ML PREPARED ENGLISH MUSTARD AND 5 ML BALSAMIC VINEGAR.
● ADD 3 THINLY SLICED MUSHROOMS BEFORE BRINGING TO THE BOIL.
● ADD 20 ML WHITE OR SOFT BROWN SUGAR, FOR A PUDDING SAUCE.

References

Cataldo, C, Debruyne, L and Witney, E. *Nutrition and Diet Therapy: Principles and Practice.* West, 5th edition, 1999

Mahan, L K and Escott-Stump, S (eds.). *Krause's Food Nutrition and Diet Therapy.* Saunders, 10th edition, 2000

150

Index